SLOW FOOD NATION

CARLO PETRINI

SLOW FOOD NATION

WHY OUR FOOD SHOULD BE GOOD, CLEAN, AND FAIR

Translated by Clara Furlan and Jonathan Hunt

Foreword by Alice Waters

Rizzoli
ex libris

First published in the United States of America in 2007
by Rizzoli Ex Libris,
an imprint of Rizzoli International Publications, Inc.
300 Park Avenue South
New York, NY 10010
www.rizzoliusa.com

Originally published in Italian in 2005 as
Buono, Pulito e Giusto by Gli struzzi Einaudi.

© 2005 Slow Food Editore srl, Bra, Italy

2013 2014 2015 2016 / 10 9 8 7 6 5 4 3 2 1

Distributed in the U.S. trade by Random House, New York

Printed in the United States of America

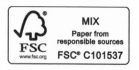

Inside pages printed on recycled paper with soy-based inks

ISBN-13: 978-0-8478-4130-1

Library of Congress Catalog Control Number: 2013931306

The aims of this book are to develop ideas, raise awareness, and arouse passion. If those aims have been achieved, much of the merit will be due to Carlo Bogliotti, who in recent years has discussed these ideas with me and rendered valuable assistance in the drafting of the text. I would like to express my gratitude to him for his generous help.

CONTENTS

FOREWORD

Alice Waters

When my friends and I opened the doors of our new restaurant Chez Panisse in 1971, we thought of ourselves as agents of seduction whose mission it was to change the way people ate. We were reacting against the uniformity and blandness of the food of the day. We soon discovered that the best-tasting food came from local farmers, ranchers, foragers, and fishermen who were committed to sound and sustainable practices. Years later, meeting Carlo Petrini for the first time, I realized that we had been a Slow Food restaurant from the start. Like Carlo, we were trying to connect pleasure and politics—by delighting our customers we could get them to pay attention to the politics of food.

Carlo Petrini is the founder of the Slow Food movement and an astonishing visionary. Unlike me, he grew up in a part of the world with a deeply traditional way of eating and living, where he learned an abiding love for the simple, life-affirming pleasures of the table. When he saw this way of eating in Italy start to disappear, he decided to do something about it. Slow Food began as an ad hoc protest against fast-food restaurants in Rome, but it has grown into an international movement built on the principles he sets forth in these pages.

Carlo has put big ideas together in sparkling, strong language that has survived translation from his robust Italian and that breathes easily and naturally. His voice is, above all, that of a person whose senses are expertly attuned, and whose mind is in constant exercise. It is a voice that is also irresistibly engaging. His argument has both the warm familial resonance of your favorite uncle's storytelling and the bracing intellectual rigor of your most inspiring teacher; its tone—now high, now low; now dry, now droll—is that of the calm and hopeful voice of reason itself. You will like this voice.

Most Americans are put off by the word gastronomy; it evokes either gastroenterology or, at best, gourmet pretention. But Carlo heroically appropriates and redefines the word.

By gastronomy he wants us to understand a new science, which he defines as the study of our food and all the natural and man-made systems that produce it. It is therefore nothing less than the study of our place on earth and our survival as a species. It is a science far more comprehensive than any of the traditional social sciences. Indeed, because gastronomy relates to the study of every subject taught in school, it can organize and enliven the curriculum as no other subject can. And if economics is the dismal science, gastronomy is certainly the cheerful one—because of its assertion of a universal right to pleasure.

The vision he sets forth in these pages is of the planet as an ark shared by all its inhabitants. The lifeline with which Carlo would bring us aboard is woven from three conceptual strands. He argues that, at every level, our food supply must meet the three criteria of quality, purity, and justice. Our food must be *buono, pulito, e giusto*—words that resonate with more solemnity in Italian than do their literal English counterparts. Our food should be *good*, and tasty to eat; it should be *clean*, produced in ways that are humane and environmentally sound; and the system by which our food is provided must be economically and socially *fair* to all who labor in it. Carlo's great insight is that when we seek out food that meets these criteria, we are no longer mere consumers but *co-producers*, who are bearing our fair share of the costs of producing good food and creating responsible communities.

Carlo's argument moves gracefully (not surprisingly, he is a very good dancer) in a way that transforms his curiosity, delight, and outrage into something like a cross between a tango and a treasure hunt. Carlo persuades us that it is the education of our senses that allows us to experience the beauty and meaning around us in the world. Few thinkers have been able to convey the delight of enlightenment so well. Carlo argues that such enlightenment can be available to every person on the planet. Thanks to his generosity and humanity and his disarming charm, it is an argument that never becomes hortatory or strident. Above all, it is the argument I have been waiting for, an irrefutable demonstration that making the right decisions about food can change the world.

INTRODUCTION

There are still people who dismiss gastronomes like me as a bunch of selfish gluttons who couldn't care less about the world around them. They misunderstand: it is precisely the gastronome's skills—which range from a finely tuned sense of taste (a skill that has deep implications for our odorless and tasteless world) to knowledge of food production—that make him care very much about the world around him, make him feel that he is in a sense a co-producer of food, a participant in a *shared destiny*.

This common destiny becomes all the clearer if we bear in mind that all human beings live on the same earth and take their nourishment from it. So this book will begin with a survey of the world's present perilous state of health, which is mainly due to the systems by which food is produced and consumed.

So, too, the new gastronome must assert his expertise in the analysis of these systems. Drawing on his long experience in the quest for the good, for culinary pleasure, he discovers that there is also a different world of production and consumption, parallel to the currently dominant one, which contains the seeds of a better global system.

However, gastronomic science and the skills that derive from it have always been misunderstood, maligned, and marginalized for a variety of reasons—this is partly the gastronome's own fault, as we shall see. So mere assertion will not be sufficient: we will have to redefine gastronomic science, give it the dignity it deserves, a new dignity. In attempting to do this in the next section of the book—an attempt that begins with a historical analysis and ends with a reasoned definition of a "new gastronomy"—the gastronome will cover the whole range of disciplines in this complex subject. He will make no claim to omniscience; indeed, he will not hesitate to call on the aid of anyone who can help him.

At this point, before moving on to the everyday act of eating, he will have to erect some fences and try to find some common factors that underlie the diversity (biological, cultural, geographical, religious, and productive) of complex gastronomy: above all, a new and precise definition of *quality*—good, clean, and fair. It is a simple definition for a very complex concept: three interdependent, essential criteria for judging the acceptability of any particular food.

Once that has been achieved, the gastronome will be able to start discussing commitments: the necessity to keep learning, to respect traditional knowledge and heed its teachings, to feel that he is a new kind of individual, what we might call a "co-producer." The co-producer/gastronome shares ideas and knowledge, shares in the quest for quality and in the quest for happiness, for a new dignity for the countryside and the people who produce food. The gastronome shares his *essence as a gastronome*—shares it with other co-producers, with producers, with chefs, and with anyone who is involved in complex gastronomy in any way; together, they all share the dual principle which is summed up in two fundamental statements (which will be explained later): "eating is an agricultural act" and "producing must be a gastronomical act."

This sharing will open people's eyes to an important sector of society which has been underestimated and ignored because it is not in line with the dominant mentality—a sector of society made up of true gastronomes (according to the new definition that I will give) who wish to build and change reality. And if that is what we all want, why not follow a plan? Why not pool our forces?

So I will end the book by discussing the idea of a *network of gastronomes* embracing the same values and commitments for all, but including a range of completely different human experiences. This network draws strength from its very diversity and may perhaps succeed in making the world a better place, or at least in improving the quality of our food and our lives. It will do so by sticking to principles that are not a mere display of good intentions, but a genuine desire to work for the *common good*. Today, this good is the most important of all causes, a source from which we can draw prosperity for ourselves and for future generations, in a world that seems to be drifting aimlessly.

If we summarize the main points of our project, this book may not appear to be too utopian:

- the gastronome examines the problems that are currently afflicting the world and traces their causes to the food system;

- the gastronome asserts his ability to interpret and influence this system through a complex science, which he *thirsts* for and which he wants others to share in as much as possible, for he is not omniscient and cannot cope with this complexity on his own;

- the gastronome demands a quality which is recognizable to all and which can improve our lives—the lives of all of us, for he cannot exist in isolation; he educates himself with others, learns from and acquires knowledge from others, exchanges with others, enjoys together with others, and feels solidarity with others.

- the gastronome will find that many others in the world share his principles and are *united* by the same desire. To join forces, to make those forces readily available to all, is the most natural thing to do in order to ensure survival and happiness for himself and his fellows. To change the world a little, since he is not the only person who wants to do so, not the only person who *hungers* for change.

I would like to end this introduction with a final thought: that phrase "to change the world a little" should be taken together with a Piedmontese expression, *per si quatr dí che 'ruma da vivi*, "for these four days that are granted to us on this earth." For these four days that are granted to us on this earth, can we not be generous? Generous to ourselves, by practicing honest pleasure; generous to those who strive to do some good in this world; and generous to all the other people, who cannot but share in our destiny?

The improvident, in the face of their "four days," do not give much thought to the future, to what will happen after they have gone. They consume, burn up, destroy, and enjoy as much as they can without a thought for the common good.

I am convinced that during these days that are granted to us on this earth—a mere moment in the history of humankind—we should try to live happily and humbly and work as hard as we can, in the healthy conviction that during those days we really do have a chance, each in our own small way, to contribute to the building of a happier future.

CHAPTER I

A WORRYING PICTURE

In each chapter I will insert some sections that I have called, for the sake of convenience, Diaries. These consist of first-person accounts of some of my experiences. I have included them because these episodes provide concrete examples of the various theories I shall try to develop in this book, and because I find that a complex subject like gastronomy must also make use of firsthand knowledge, of traveling, and of direct contact with other cultures or with one's own roots. You cannot become a gastronome simply by reading books: you need to put your theories into practice; you must be curious, you must try to read reality with your senses, by coming into contact with as many different environments as possible, by talking to people, and by tasting. You cannot become a gastronome simply by eating in restaurants; you must meet the small farmers, the people who produce and process food, the people who strive to make the production-consumption system fairer, to render it sustainable and enjoyable.

Thanks to my work, I have been lucky enough to have had many such experiences, and each of them has had a strong influence on my own development and on the evolution of the ideas that you will encounter. I enjoy telling these stories; I find it useful for the purposes of the book, and I am sure the reader will understand the reasons behind their inclusion.

In effect, these episodes are like phases in a journey through life and through thought: I am indebted to them, and to the people involved in them, for a large part of the content of this book.

In 1996, I happened to be traveling, as I often do, along
the SS (*strada statale*, or state highway) 231, which links
Cuneo with Asti, passing via Bra, the small provincial town
where I live and where the international movement Slow
Food is based. Even today, although a highway is being
built to connect the two larger towns, this busy strip of
asphalt running across southern Piedmont is virtually our
only link with the rest of Italy. It runs in an easterly direction, and anyone who wishes to travel toward Milan or
central and southern Italy is bound to use it.

Southern Piedmont has always been an agricultural
region; its history has included many periods of hunger
and deprivation, but more recently the area has been
enriched by the introduction of small industries and by the
emergence of a mutually beneficial interchange between
the area's traditional agricultural wares—including some
of the finest of all Italian wines—and burgeoning international tourism. As the production and export of local gastronomic treasures has grown, tourists have been drawn
not just by the beauty of southern Piedmont's hilly landscape, but by its gastronomy, too.

The SS 231 runs across this countryside and, as well
as being notorious for its inadequacies as a thoroughfare, it
has become a striking symbol of the affluence that has
transformed the land of my birth. It runs along a long
string of factories, suburban shopping centers, and big-box
stores that are among the worst architectural horrors that
could possibly be imagined. Only here and there do you
still find a few surviving greenhouses where things are
grown. It is a depressing experience to drive through such
squalid surroundings, especially as the slowness of the
road always gives you plenty of time to meditate at length
on "development" and its effects.

Along the road—if you make just the smallest of
detours—the concentration of excellent restaurants and

traditional *osterie* serving local cuisine is far higher than in any other part of Italy. It was here that I began to learn about gastronomy, and I owe a crucial part of my training as a gastronome to the chefs and farmers of this area.

But to return to that day in 1996: on my way home, I stopped at a restaurant owned by a friend of mine whom I hadn't seen for several years and who was renowned for his *peperonata* (a common Italian dish whose Piedmont version is traditionally made with the "square" peppers of Asti). I wanted to have a helping of his specialty to refresh myself after the tiring journey that was now nearing its end; to my great disappointment, the *peperonata* I was served was awful—completely tasteless. The chef's skills were not in doubt, so I asked for an explanation for this great deterioration in flavor. My friend told me that he no longer used the same raw materials as those of the *peperonata* that echoed in my gustatory-olfactory memory. The square peppers of Asti, a fleshy, scented, tasty variety, had almost ceased to be grown locally, so instead he used peppers imported from Holland—imported because they were cheaper, grown with intensive farming methods, using hybrid varieties that were visually striking with their garish colors, and perfect for export ("each box contains thirty-two peppers, not one more, not one less, and every one beautiful, every one identical," he told me). But they were utterly tasteless.

Resigned to the fact that the wonderful *peperonata* had gone forever, I drove on down the road toward Bra. Passing along one of the stretches of road where there are still some greenhouses, I stopped the car at a place called Costigliole d'Asti: surely this was where they used to grow those square Asti peppers? What could be under those nylon sheets now? I met a farmer, who confirmed that it was indeed here that those magnificent vegetables had been grown. But not anymore; as he explained to me: "It's not worth it: the Dutch ones are cheaper and nobody buys ours any longer. It's hard work producing them and it's all wasted effort." "What do you grow now, then?" I asked. He smiled: "Tulip bulbs! And after we've grown the bulbs, we send them to Holland where they bring them into bloom."

I was dumbfounded. I had come up against one of the paradoxes of agroindustry and its interaction with globalization: peppers crossing frontiers and traveling over mountains in exchange for tulips; products that were the symbols of two different regions being grown more than a thousand kilometers away from their respective homes, completely overturning the two agricultural traditions that had once firmly embedded them in their original ecosystems; a wonderful variety of pepper now on the verge of extinction; a traditional recipe distorted out of all recognition; and goodness knows how much pollution from fertilizers and pesticides and from exhaust fumes discharged into the air by container trucks and other vehicles going back and forth across Europe.

That day for me was the official starting date of *ecogastronomy*: the raw material must be grown and produced in a sustainable way; biodiversity and local traditions of cuisine and production must be preserved even if it costs more.

....

{DIARY 2} TEHUACÁN
....

During the summer of 2001, I went on a trip, first to San Francisco, to attend the First National Congress of Slow Food USA, then on to Mexico, a country and a culture of which I am very fond and which I had not visited for some time. I stayed for a while in the Federal District of the immense Mexico City, where I saw with my own eyes the extreme poverty endured by millions of people who had left the countryside, selling off what little land they possessed, and who were now clogging up the suburbs of the capital in the hope of making a living. The small-scale, family-based subsistence farming they practiced was no longer profitable: the neighboring United States had created illusions with the glitter of its products and stimulated new needs, but its primary effect had been to impose the methods of industrial farming. The latter had reduced the workforce, made it difficult to avoid being drawn into the vicious circle imposed by the multinationals (the commercialization of seeds, fertilizers, and pesticides—all interlinked products), and stripped a farming culture of its traditional knowledge, formed over thousands of years.

In Mexico, where the pre-Columbian civilizations were responsible for developing corn and many other food products that are now part of the basic diet of millions of people around the world, biodiversity is still at record levels. As far as corn is concerned, of the more than a thousand indigenous varieties that evolved over the centuries in perfect harmony with the various Mexican ecosystems, I was told that over the years almost 80 percent have been patented by American multinationals searching for new hybrids.

These local varieties have then been gradually replaced by those very same American hybrids, which need much more water (and many parts of Mexico suffer from a serious water shortage), as well as having a far lower nutritional value and poorer taste. Tortillas made with corn soaked in water with a little lime (the presence of so much calcium in such a widespread dish meant that dental problems were almost unknown in Mexico until fifty years ago) were—and to some extent still are—a homemade product, skillfully cooked by the women and rich in flavors which vary according to the type of corn used. This gastronomic richness should not be underestimated: together with the infinite variety of traditional Indian cuisines, which were always based on local products, it has made Mexican gastronomy one of the most complex in the world. (Much of the country's rich gastronomic heritage has been documented by José N. Iturriaga de la Fuente, a winner of the 2003 Slow Food award for the defense of biodiversity.)[1]

The spread of the intensive cultivation of corn has threatened other vegetable species, too, such as amaranth. This food, together with beans and corn, was the basis of the Aztec diet, but was banned by the first colonizers because it was felt to be in some way associated with the ritual human sacrifices that these civilizations practiced. As a result, it has become extremely rare, gradually forgotten by the local farming cultures, and this is a pity, for not only does the plant need very little water to complete its productive cycle, but it also constitutes an ideal supplement to the country dwellers' poor diet.[2]

So that summer I went to Tehuacán, in the state of Puebla, to learn more about an excellent project—winner of the 2002 Slow Food Award for the Defense of Biodiversity—to reintroduce amaranth to one of the poorest areas in Mexico, where the desert is inexorably advancing. The Quali project, founded and directed by Raúl Hernández Garciadiego, is combined with an ingenious plan to regenerate the water supply using some clever methods devised by the ancient inhabitants of this area.

I visited a tiny family-run farm to see a small amaranth allotment with my own eyes and to hear from the farmers themselves what they thought of the project. With me went the directors of Quali, some of my own colleagues, and Alicia De Angeli, a well-known Mexico City chef and an expert on native Mexican cuisines, which she skillfully recreates in her own restaurant.

The poverty of the family we met was unmistakable, but they were very dignified and expressed satisfaction at having found a plant, the amaranth, that was easier to grow and more profitable than corn. Their house was modest; the children played on a small threshing floor strewn with disused tools, fragments of Coca-Cola bottles, and empty Pan Bimbo wrappers. (Pan Bimbo, the best-known brand of bread produced by the Mexican food industry, is gradually supplanting corn tortillas in the everyday diet of the poorer sectors of society, creating many nutritional problems in a country where white bread made from wheat had never formed part of the traditional diet.)

The little amaranth field was close to the farm buildings, and as we walked back to the farmhouse after viewing those colorful plants, I overheard an interesting conversation between De Angeli and the wife of the farmer who was our host. The two women stopped by the side of the short path down which we were walking. There were weeds all along the path; in fact, the house was completely surrounded by weeds. The attention of the two women (both of them cooks, but very different from one another, and it was a striking visual contrast to see them together— the one white and of European origin, a member of the affluent elite of the Federal District; the other a poor native Mexican, her spine curved by constant physical labor) was attracted to one of these leafy weeds. "This is a wonderful herb! But I'm sure you know it, don't you?" De Angeli asked. "No, why?" said the lady of the house. "It's excellent for making *caldos* [broths and soups]; they're very nutritious, and tasty, too. The recipes I discovered during my research originate from this very area; they're traditional to your people." The perplexity of this farmer's wife, a woman of about forty, was shyly expressed on her face as she asked the white chef for an explanation of how to make soup with that plant. De Angeli meticulously explained the recipes.

We visited the kitchen. The limited range of utensils and of food in the pantry spoke volumes about how difficult it was for these people to find enough food to put on their plates day by day. The house was surrounded by freely growing herbs that over the centuries their ancestors had learned to use for nutritional and medicinal purposes, but they themselves had no idea how to cook them; in fact, they weren't even aware that they were edible.

Industrial agriculture and modernization wiped the slate clean: all it took was the introduction of a few cultivable varieties of the most common products—varieties which do not thrive in this increasingly arid environment—and within two generations the local population had lost all the traditional knowledge that had once enabled it to subsist on the freely available fruits of nature. A simple form of gastronomic knowledge, an ancient wisdom, a recipe, had disappeared from local culture and made life even more difficult in this region where the temptation to sell your field and move to Mexico City, or to take a job in the nearby *maquiladoras* making jeans for American firms, is stronger than anywhere else in the country.

Evening was falling in Tehuacán. Just as we reached the threshing floor, the truck that makes door-to-door deliveries of Pan Bimbo stopped at the end of the street, under a huge billboard advertising Coca-Cola, the American company which, ironically, owns the largest spring of bottled mineral water in Mexico, itself called Tehuacán. Even today, Tehuacán is synonymous for bottled water all over Mexico; in many parts of the country, it is the standard term that people use when ordering mineral water in bars. The factory that bottles it stood out on the skyline a few kilometers from our friends' house, in this stretch of land which is among the thirstiest and driest in Central America.

. . . .

{**DIARY 3**} LAGUIOLE
. . . .

In the late spring of 2001, a business trip took me to France: to Lyon and Laguiole. I was due to have a couple of meetings with the local directors of Slow Food France in the regional capital and make a stopover in Aubrac, an area south of the Massif Central, bordering on the more famous Auvergne. There, in the principal village of the area, Laguiole, I was to meet André Valadier, the president of the Jeune Montagne cooperative, which produces Laguiole cheese, one of the many French cheeses classified as Appellation d'Origine Contrôlée (AOC). I should explain that Laguiole not only denotes a village and a cheese, but is probably even more famous as the name of a traditional knife, a minor art form which is considered the knife *par excellence* by all French gourmets.

Valadier is a very charismatic figure, the head of the association of AOC cheese producers, and I wanted to meet him to discuss the possibility of their attending Cheese, the international conference which Slow Food holds every two years in Bra, in September.

The visit also gave me an excuse to dine and stay at one of the most charming and relaxing *relais* in France, that of Michel Bras, a three-star chef based in Laguiole. He is a close friend of Valadier and a great champion of regional cuisine and local biodiversity: in his recipes he uses more than three hundred kinds of vegetables, from the most common to the very rarest, and from cultivated varieties to others that grow wild in the vast pastures and woods of the beautiful Aubrac plateau.

Between a quick meeting in the afternoon, in the offices of Jeune Montagne, and a wonderful dinner *chez* Bras, Valadier recounted to me the history of Laguiole (the cheese) and of this region, which for geomorphological reasons is somewhat isolated from the rest of France.

"Until World War II," Valadier told me, "we produced cheese mainly for our own sustenance. Later, we strove to produce as much as possible, and today we've reached the point where we have to produce in order to have a surplus."

In the 1960s, the Aubrac, like almost all the mountain areas of Europe, entered a period of profound social and productive crisis. First came emigration: the young rejected the harsh conditions demanded by agricultural life and left for the cities, abandoning the care of pastures, the raising of the local breed of cattle—the Fleur d'Aubrac (or Rouge d'Aubrac)—and the production of cheese. The few who remained, of whom Valadier was one, were persuaded by zootechnical experts to switch from local breeds of cattle to Holsteins, the famous dappled black-and-white creatures that invaded the world milk market in the late 1970s. They are the most productive of all cows: they stand quietly in their stables, pumped with feed specially formulated to squeeze every last drop out of them. When they reach the end of their "careers," they are fattened up as quickly as possible—in America through hormones, in Europe until recently with the animal flour that caused mad cow disease—and then sent to the abattoir. Since, owing to the life they have led, their meat is not particularly good, they are mainly used for hamburgers or other industrial products.[3] But they do have one advantage, at first sight: they produce almost twice as much milk per day as "normal" cows.

The Aubrac farmers could hardly believe it when they were shown those production figures. Within a few years, Holsteins had replaced the Aubrac cows almost to the point of rendering them extinct. Problems, however, soon began to arise: the Holsteins, because of their physical characteristics, are not suited to grazing on high ground, and in the Aubrac, with all those pastures, cattle sheds are almost pointless, except to shelter the animals from the winter cold. Moreover, their milk, which contains much less fat and also less protein than that produced by the indigenous cows (as well as being less tasty), is virtually useless for making Laguiole cheese, whose traditional production method requires milk with very different characteristics. So, along with the indigenous cows, the traditional cheese was also disappearing.

And as if this were not enough, emigration had led to the expertise in knife production moving to Thiers, where there are some big firms specializing in that sector.

The three symbols of Laguiole—grazing cattle, cheese, and knives—were on the point of being erased from history in the space of twenty years.

"I decided that it was time to start a campaign," said Valadier. "I set up a cooperative with some other young people who had not left the area, and we pinned our hopes on the few remaining Fleur d'Aubrac cows. Since then, there have been a lot of changes: now you can again see in the pastures our reddish-brown cows with those black circles round their eyes and those long, downward-turned horns that are used for making knife handles. Now you are sitting here in front of me in one of the finest restaurants in France, inviting me to bring Laguiole to Bra for Cheese, and you have asked me for the address of a place where you can buy a set of knives for your sister. I'd say that we have achieved results here, wouldn't you?"

The next day, while I was paying a considerable price—but a fair one, I must admit, all things considered—for the knives I wanted to take home with me, I pondered those words. During my homeward journey, through those pastures that form such a breathtaking landscape, I thought of the many other mountainous regions of Europe, of the pastures that had run wild, of the ghost villages, of the cheeses that needed protection because they were on the verge of extinction, of the landslides, of the increasingly frequent floods, and of the woods that had turned into thickets. I thought of the productivism of the "milk machine," and of the Holsteins.

....

1. A WORRYING PICTURE

The Diaries that introduced this first short chapter illustrate three of the typical situations that have arisen in the world of farming and food production since World War II. They are three snapshots of the social, economic, and cultural changes that occurred in the second half of the twentieth century, a transformation unprecedented in human history.

I must ask my readers to be patient, because this chapter describes a situation about which they will already have heard, but although my remarks are not completely new, I consider them an essential prelude to what will follow. The gastronomic perspective cannot ignore these questions, and they must be clearly explained at the outset so that we can understand their links with gastronomic science and appreciate how a correct application of certain principles in the field of nutrition can bring benefits in the future.

To return to the situations described in the first three Diaries of this book, the side effects of the process of industrialization that has swept through the world during the past two centuries are clear. First, it has significantly improved the quality of life of millions of people—almost all of whom live in what is usually described as the Western hemisphere—generating what is commonly termed "development." For example, in many parts of the world, malnutrition and difficulty in obtaining food have become distant memories. All this "development," however, has proved to have great limitations and has created a number of situations which, in this age of globalization, the postindustrial age, the world system seems unlikely to be able to tolerate for much longer—situations, in short, which are *unsustainable*.

Along with the process of industrialization, in little more than a century a kind of technocratic dictatorship has been established, where profit prevails over politics and economics over culture, and where quantity is the main, if not the sole, criterion for judging human activities. Edgar Morin, the French philosopher, sociologist, and theorist of complexity, has spoken of "four engines" that drive "spaceship Earth": four interconnected engines which produce "blind and ever-accelerating progress." The four engines are science, technology, industry, and the capitalist economy.[4] These four engines are both invasive and pervasive, for the process of industrialization did not stop at manufactured articles and consumer products, but has entered, as a cultural factor, into the daily life of human beings, conditioning every activity.

The four engines have imposed a totalitarian regime where technology and economics have the upper hand—where they become the sole purpose rather than a means for serving the aims and values of the community. This is an absolute predominance which feeds on globalization and spreads with it, becoming in turn the main standardizing factor for the whole world. All this is happening with increasing speed, because the main objective now seems to be the reduction of time to zero, according to Jérôme Bindé, assistant to the director general for the social and human sciences and director of the Forecasting, Philosophy, and Human Sciences division of UNESCO:

> Where will it all end? The times we are living in today are entirely dominated by what I call "the tyranny of urgency" both in the financial field, where transactions are now made in a fraction of a second, and in the media, the realm of the ephemeral, or even on the political scene, where the next election seems the only temporal horizon of public action. Our societies live in a kind of instantaneanism which prevents them from controlling the future.[5]

The supremacy of technology thus creates a new ideology, which denies and conceals the complexity of the world and of the relations and interdependencies that characterize it, and also their value, tempting us to make the mistake of trying to analyze it in a linear manner, when this is not in fact possible.

Moreover, "linear" values, such as progress, the control of nature, and a rationality that tends to quantify everything, obliterate what were once described as differences in class, while widening the gap between civilizations: between a West that has "developed" on the basis of those values and the rest of the world, which seems to be crushed by the West's dominant principles and given a simple, inevitable, and agonizing choice between outright refusal or acceptance and "alignment." But the choice is important only in a relative sense, for it has always led to more or less obvious manifestations of what has been termed a new form of colonization.

2. A SINGLE DESTINY: NATURE, MAN, AND FOOD

The men and women of the world perform complex productive activities conditioned by centuries of culture and know-how— activities that are representations of diversities and identities, the products of relations and social interdependencies, mirrors of the complexity of the world. These human activities are strongly influenced by the relationship between man and nature, an intimate connection which has changed radically since the rise of industrial capitalism.

Nature has become an object of domination, and we can see the effects of this if we consider what has been done in the so-called food and agriculture sector. At the end of World War II, in response to the needs of a hungry world, this sector underwent a complete transformation, immediately adhering to the techno-cratic ideology. Agriculture, a source of food for humanity, had to assume the colors, characteristics, and dimensions of the classic industrial sector, turning into what is commonly termed *agro-industry*: an unfortunate term that conceals a number of contra-dictions. In fact, it is an oxymoron.

Today, we are still paying for this and other major transfor-mations at a price that is unsustainable for the planet. Economic theories have tried to introduce the concept of *negative externali-ties,*[6] in order to quantify the collateral damage that the "four engines" have done to society: pollution, soil death, the scarring of landscapes, the reduction of energy sources, and the loss of diver-sity, both biological (biodiversity) and cultural. But it is still diffi-cult to reduce such complex problems to a linear calculation, to quantify all the possible environmental, social, and cultural costs (the fact they are termed *externalities* is an indication of how little consideration they have been given, except as a phenomenon external to industrial processes). In the meantime, all we can do is count the casualties, or simply accept that "spaceship Earth" is heading for disaster. It is no longer a secret or a claim of the more radical environmentalists: we consume more than it is possible for the planet to provide without upsetting its own equilibrium.

3. THE MILLENNIUM ASSESSMENT

The Millennium Ecosystem Assessment was commissioned in 2000 by United Nations Secretary-General Kofi Annan in order to study the impact of ecosystem change on human health and to document the actions needed to help conserve ecosystems. Its report was published in March 2005, after four years of work by 1,360 experts from a variety of organizations, including the Food and Agriculture Organization (FAO) and the World Wide Fund for Nature (WWF). Writing about the report's publication, journalist Antonio Cianciullo adopted this very appropriate metaphor:

> We are facing ecological bankruptcy and our first possessions are already being pawned: during the last twenty-five years we have seen one in three mangrove forests and one in five coral barriers disappear; two out of every three ecosystems are showing signs of decline; 25 percent of mammals, 12 percent of birds, and 32 percent of amphibians are threatened with extinction.[7]

That is, indeed, a very serious picture, and it led the director general of the Food and Agriculture Organization, Jacques Diouf, to speak of "mortgaging the future" and of "thresholds of mass extinction":

> Over the past fifty years, humans have changed ecosystems more rapidly and extensively than in any comparable period of time in human history, largely to meet rapidly growing demands for food, fresh water, timber, fiber, and fuel. This has resulted in a substantial and largely irreversible loss in the diversity of life on Earth.[8]

The loss is being incurred by what is commonly called *biodiversity*, or, according to the definition given at the Earth Summit held at Rio de Janeiro in 1992:

> the variability among living organisms from all sources including, inter alia, terrestrial, marine, and other aquatic

ecosystems and the ecological complexes of which they are part; this includes diversity within species, between species, and of ecosystems.[9]

According to the Millennium Assessment, the situation is mainly due to a massive conversion of land to agricultural use: since 1945, there have been more land occupations than in the two previous centuries, and today cultivated land occupies a quarter of the surface of the planet. Water consumption has doubled since 1960, and 70 percent of it is used in agriculture. Over the same period, the emission of nitrates into the ecosystems has doubled and that of phosphates has tripled. Over half the amount of chemical fertilizers that have ever been produced—since their invention at the turn of the twentieth century—have been used in the years since 1985. The concentration of carbon dioxide in the atmosphere has risen by 32 percent since 1750, mainly because of the use of fossil fuels and changes in land use (such as deforestation). About 60 percent of this increase has occurred since 1959.

Such a level of interference in the balance of nature has significantly reduced biological diversity around the world: during the last hundred years, the coefficient of species extinction has increased a thousandfold compared with the average over the whole history of our planet. Genetic diversity has undergone a global decline, especially as far as cultivated species are concerned.

As stated in the synthesis of the Millennium Assessment, these changes in the ecosystem

> have contributed to substantial net gains in human well-being and economic development, but these gains have been achieved at growing costs in the form of the degradation of many ecosystem services, increased risks of nonlinear changes, and the exacerbation of poverty for some groups of people. These problems, unless addressed, will substantially diminish the benefits that future generations obtain from ecosystems.[10]

It must be said that one of the benefits obtained from ecosystems, and the most important and irreplaceable of them all, is nutrition. The most significant changes have been made in response to the growing demand for food and water: agriculture, fishing, and harvesting have been the main factors in all the strategies of "development."

Between 1960 and 2000, the world population doubled, while food production rose by two and a half times. Today, there are six billion people in the world, and according to the Food and Agriculture Organization, current food production is sufficient for twelve billion people. In the face of these figures, is it still legitimate to speak of "development"?

4. RESTORING FOOD TO ITS CENTRAL PLACE

Food production is rising, the amount of cultivated land is increasing, and 22 percent of the world population (almost half of the total workforce) is engaged in agriculture, but the food produced for twelve billion people is in fact not enough to feed the six billion who actually live in the world. Moreover, this effort of production has not achieved its aims. It has subjected the earth to such stress that the land either succumbs to desertification or dies because of the excessive use of chemical products. Water resources are running out. Biodiversity is rapidly diminishing, especially agro-biodiversity, with a continual reduction in the number of animal breeds and vegetable varieties that have for centuries contributed to the sustenance of entire regions in a perfectly sustainable alliance between man and nature.

Something must have gone wrong, because if we consider the problem of satisfying the primal need for food and analyze it over the long term, the hunger for production has done more harm than good.

The contradiction in agroindustrial terms is clearly emerging: agroindustry has given us the illusion that it could solve the problem of feeding the human race. I would go even further: over the last fifty years, it has turned food production into both executioner and victim. Executioner, because the unsustainable methods of agroindustry have led to the disappearance of many sustainable production methods which were once part of the identity of the communities that practiced them and were one of the highest pleasures for the gastronome in search of valuable knowledge and flavors. Victim, because the same unsustainable methods—originally necessary in order to feed a larger number of people—have since turned the sphere of food and agriculture into a neglected sector, completely detached from the lives of billions of people, as if procuring food had become a matter of course and required no effort at all. Politics shows little interest in it, except when pressured to do so by the most powerful lobbies of international agroindustry, while the average consumer either does not reflect on what he or she is eating or has to make a titanic effort to obtain the information that will explain it.

Food and its production must regain the central place that they deserve among human activities, and we must reexamine the criteria that guide our actions. The crucial point now is no longer, as it has been for all too long, the quantity of food that is produced, but its complex quality, a concept that ranges from the question of taste to that of variety, from respect for the environment, the ecosystems, and the rhythms of nature to respect for human dignity. The aim is to make a significant improvement to everybody's quality of life without having to submit, as we have done until now, to a model of development that is incompatible with the needs of the planet.

5. AGROINDUSTRY?

It should be stated at the outset that if food is to regain its central place, we will have to concern ourselves with agriculture. It is impossible to discuss food without discussing agriculture. Every gastronome should be aware of this, because the present situation in the world is the result of the history of Western agriculture (and the damage it has done to nature), an agriculture that has lost sight of some of the aims that are most important to anyone who cares about the quality of food.

This history tells us above all of an exponential rise in productivity. The process began slowly, in the second half of the eighteenth century, with the introduction of leguminous and fodder plants into the crop rotation. This was a revolutionary development that allowed the soil to refertilize more effectively and rapidly than in the past, and always—it should be emphasized—in a natural way. At the same time, it gave a boost to stock farming. The result was a general rise in production, which increased even more when elements external to the natural cycle of an agricultural ecosystem began to be introduced: first organic refuse from nearby towns, then the boom in Peruvian guano and other organic fertilizers imported from ever more distant places. Later, when these resources were either running out or were no longer sufficient on their own, came the great invention of chemical fertilizers produced on an industrial scale. If we consider these changes in terms of naturalness, we cannot fail to notice that there has been a gradual but continual (and increasingly rapid) trend toward *unnaturalness*.

The formulas of chemical fertilizers were first developed in the 1840s, and they have been the crucial factor in the escalation of modern industrial agriculture and its unnaturalness.[11] The trend toward chemistry did not just carry on the tradition of introducing elements alien to the existing ecosystems, but introduced inorganic elements that it ended up overusing. During the past twenty years, we have used more than twice as many chemical fertilizers as we had ever previously produced! Can the earth sustain such a change in its balance?

As Debal Deb stated in a 2004 publication, modern agricultural and forestry sciences have created a simplification and homogenization of nature in order to minimize uncertainty and to ensure an efficient production of commercial goods: agriculture today consists of an intensification of a few crops, to the detriment of a magnificent genetic diversity created through millennia of experimentation. The monocultures of those varieties that are valid from the commercial point of view have shaped modern agriculture, which works as a means of rapidly eliminating life forms, impoverishing the soil, and destroying the systems that support life on earth. The worst thing, Deb goes on to say, is that, despite the plethora of empirical evidence on the adverse consequences of large-scale industrial agriculture, this has become the model to follow for agricultural development in all the countries that try to emulate the Western model of growth.[12]

The absurd idea (it is a contradiction in terms!) of *industrial agriculture*—agriculture carried out according to the principles of industry—is thus dominant. Under industrial agriculture, the fruits of nature are considered raw materials to be consumed and processed on a mass scale. The subversion of the natural order has affected the entire food production system. The agroindustry of food production has become the model of development in a world in which technology reigns. And if it has done enormous damage in the Western world which invented it, the imposition of a single method of development based on technocratic thought has created even worse problems elsewhere. It has done untold harm to the environments and people of the countries that are poorest in material wealth (though certainly not in biodiversity), and to traditions and cultures that have existed for centuries in perfect harmony with their ecosystems.

6. A NEW AGRICULTURE FOR THE PLANET

The so-called Green Revolution, which began under the aegis of the World Bank after World War II, shed a ray of hope on many parts of the world that were then suffering from starvation. Fertilizers and new hybrid varieties that increased production significantly, generating more than one harvest per year, made it possible to solve the problems of nutrition in some areas of the planet; but those areas were too few, because in the final analysis the Green Revolution was an ecological and economic disaster.

I have already mentioned the significant impoverishment of natural resources due to industrial agriculture: the new hybrid varieties consume more water; they replace the existing biodiversity, permanently eliminating it; and they indirectly ruin the quality of the soil, which needs ever-increasing quantities of chemical fertilizers and pesticides.

But the disaster is even worse than this. First, in addition to the loss of biodiversity and of traditional agronomic techniques, we have lost a priceless heritage of knowledge not only about the cultivation and beneficial effects of certain plants in particular ecosystems, but also about the use, processing, and preparation of products. Moreover, since agricultural growth is rightly considered to be one of the main factors in the development of poorer countries, the Green Revolution opened up a huge new market for the operations of the big multinationals, which make most of their profits in three sectors: seeds, fertilizers, and pesticides. The power acquired by some of these gigantic concerns came to resemble a kind of colonization in developing countries, which has since taken the form of an aggressive and increasingly resented domination.

The final balance sheet is beginning to show the effects of these changes: enormous damage caused to the ecosystem; an increase in food production that has not solved the problems of hunger and malnutrition; and an incalculable loss from the cultural and social point of view. From this latter viewpoint, ancient traditions and knowledge have been discarded like the proverbial baby with the bathwater; the rural population has abandoned the countryside to clog up the cities (a phenomenon that is reaching catastrophic proportions in the developing countries, creating megalopolises like New Delhi or Mexico City); and there has been a wholesale loss of gastronomic and culinary knowledge that was once the basis of a correct—as well as enjoyable—use of agricultural resources. We are witnessing a form of cultural annihilation that has affected the countryside of every part of the world, on a scale that is unprecedented in human history.

There is therefore an urgent need for new kinds of farming, a truly *new agriculture*. Sustainable methods can take their starting point from the small (or large, depending on where in the world you are) amount of knowledge that has not been eliminated by agroindustrial methods. This will not be a return to the past, but rather a new beginning that grows out of the past, with an awareness of the mistakes that have been made in recent years. It will involve making productive again those areas where agriculture has been abandoned because it was not viable according to industrial criteria; preserving, improving, and spreading the knowledge of the traditional practices which are demonstrating that other modes of production are possible; and giving new dignity and new opportunities to the people who have been marginalized by the globalization of agriculture.

Only through a new sustainable agriculture that respects both old traditions and modern technologies (for the new technologies are not bad in themselves; it all depends on how one uses them) can we begin to have hopes of a better future. And only through its diffusion will gastronomes be able to move from their present state of protesters against the prevailing trends to that of fulfilled people who still regard food as a central element in our lives.

7. THE GASTRONOME

There is a theory that man, since he is convinced that he can dominate nature and that it is entirely at his disposal, strives to find solutions through technology, but that with every technological answer he devises, he in fact creates new and more serious problems. I would say that this is true of the earth today, and we seem to have reached the absolute limit.

This situation demands much more than a simple change, of course: it demands a radical change in mentality, more complexity of thought, and more humility and a greater sense of responsibility toward nature.

The present systems of food production are among the main causes of this state of affairs and of this way of thinking, which is so strongly influenced by Western capitalist culture. Yet, at the same time, the systems of food production themselves suffer very badly from the effects of that state of affairs and of that way of thinking.

We are what we eat: this is true, and considering the present trends in the world, we are beginning to seem far more savage in our way of eating than our prehistoric ancestors. Food, and a careful study of how it is produced, sold, and consumed, is in fact a form of evidence that can open our eyes to what we have become and to where we are headed. It can enable us to sketch out an interpretation of the complex systems that govern the world and our lives and yet—this is the theory that I wish to propound—it still leaves us scope to rebuild the foundations for a sustainable future. Many of the ideas I will present have been prompted by my personal experience as a gastronome, particularly during the past twenty years since I became president of the international Slow Food movement (the Diaries at the beginning of each chapter give concrete examples of these experiences). My point of departure is the assertion of a fundamental human right which the gastronome defends: the right to pleasure, a natural, physiological right, the denial of which has contributed greatly to the present global situation. That situation is a very complicated one, but I think gastronomy can provide us with some useful keys to understanding it. Let us now examine how it can do so, starting with a reevaluation of gastronomic science, which we will redefine in modern, sustainable terms.

CHAPTER II

GASTRONOMY AND NEW GASTRONOMY

The gastronomes of my generation were inevitably self-taught. Not many wine-tasting courses existed, and there was certainly no University of Gastronomic Sciences, as there is now in Italy (see page 160). Apart from our first gastronomic experiences, our first important bottles of wine, and our first noteworthy restaurants, therefore, the main formative influences in a gastronome's life were the people who stimulated us to learn more about the subject. These people were in effect our teachers; the education they gave us was supplemented by our own private reading and by the early television cooking programs.

As far as my own experience is concerned, while I should stress that I live in a region where gastronomic subjects are part of everyday life, the people I regard as my teachers were acquaintances, writers, and television personalities, though the world they belong to has since changed considerably; in some respects, it is more aware, but in others, it is far more superficial.

I would start with Luigi Veronelli, who was probably the most important Italian food-and-wine connoisseur in the twentieth century. He was the first real pioneer of modern gastronomic literature and television in Italy. His work was particularly interesting because it had a solid scientific, historical, and philosophical basis. I have fond memories of him, because he invented a new way of talking about food and wine, because his words enriched and defined the Italian vocabulary on the subject, and because he was the first to champion the small farmers and producers, the true creators of the pleasures of the table. His guides and other books were the basis of the education of thousands of enthusiasts of my generation, and gave a crucial impulse to the growth of the Italian food-and-wine industry, making it what it is today.

On television, too, the program he copresented with Ave Ninchi was groundbreaking in the way it used the new medium to present the subject. My first great television influence, however, was Mario Soldati, a remarkable character—gastronome, poet, novelist, and film director. I remember how in 1957 my whole family was always glued to the screen when his program *Viaggio nella valle del Po. All ricerca dei cibi più genuini* (A Journey Through the Po Valley: In Search of Genuine Food) was on. In that historical production of Italian television, the far-sightedness of the poet and the great film director brought out extremely well the transition that postwar Italy was going through. It was a total transition, from an agricultural economy to an industrial one, and it led to the rise of agroindustry. Nowadays, that series is still indispensable for an understanding of the transformations that took place in Italy, as we saw in the previous chapter, and it has even more value now that a great part of that agricultural tradition has disappeared.

To turn now to those who had a direct influence on my attitudes and my mode of being, there are three key figures, all of whom were working in my region, so I was able to appreciate their human and gastronomic qualities firsthand: Bartolo Mascarello, a producer of Barolo; Battista Rinaldi, another Barolo producer and mayor of the small town that gives its name to the king of the Langhe wines; and Luciano De Giacomi, former president of the Association of the Knights of the Truffle.

Bartolo Mascarello, an unforgettable winegrower whose 2005 death was mourned not just by his family but by the many lovers of his products, personified in every way the identity of the people of the Langhe—indeed, the identity of the Langhe itself. His strong links with the area and its traditions are irreplaceable; they, together with his rigorous political and moral vision, will be his true monument. Until the last days of his life, I delighted in his company: talking to him was like talking with the land itself, sharing in its transformations and caring passionately about its conservation. His wine is that of a producer who—long before the importance of such things was recognized by others—always sought that principle of quality which I will discuss in more detail later. He gave me the first concrete example I ever saw of production according to criteria that corresponded to three fundamental principles which I will call "good, clean, and fair": respect for sensory quality, for environmental sustainability, and for the workers, the people who actually produce.

Battista Rinaldi, mayor of the small town of Barolo, was also a producer of Barolo wine. In the late 1970s, I was entranced by his recherché but agreeable way of speaking, which was a little flowery but always in keeping with his role as a true *amphitryon*, or host of formal banquets. Having been for many years not only mayor of the town but also president of the Enoteca Barolo (Barolo Wine Association), he made a name for himself as an organizer of dinners, practicing the noble art which Alexandre-Balthazar-Laurent Grimod de La Reynière had codified in his *Manuel des amphitryons* (1808). Each banquet or symposium organized by the Enoteca was preceded by one of his talks, during which he could hold his audience's attention and engage their interest in the subjects of food and the pleasure of eating better than I had ever seen anyone do. I think the *amphitryon* still has an important role in directing a banquet and putting the guests at their ease, mediating between scientific terminology and the language of gastronomic pleasure. It is a vital skill if we wish to convey information or sensations and teach people about food.

On the same wavelength was another great character from my area, Luciano De Giacomi, with whom I came into contact many years later, after a long period during which we avoided each other because he was an altogether gruffer, more demanding, and in some ways more difficult person. He was the epitome of conservative Piedmont, expecting rigor in everyday life from others, but quite consistent in making the same demands on himself. After successfully organizing the first international convention on Piedmontese wines in 1990, I was made a Friend of the Associazione dei Cavalieri del Tartufo (Association of the Knights of the Truffle), of which he was then president, and I attended many symposiums of this excellent organization. I was struck by the sternness and authority with which De Giacomi organized these events: where Rinaldi was easygoing and affable, De Giacomi was prickly and stiff. But they were two sides of the same coin, and from both of them I learned a great deal about the significance of the figure of the gastronome and how important it is for him to be able to communicate with others.

From the more strictly "gourmetistic" (if I may be pardoned the neologism) point of view, another important influence on me was Dr. Giusto Piolatto, a true connoisseur of good food whose approach to gastronomic pleasure fascinated me. He was one of the first critics of the *Guida ristoranti* (Restaurant Guide) published by the weekly magazine *Espresso*. He taught me a lot about restaurant-going and how to judge food, because his approach to pleasure was always enriched by a genuine sympathy for, and profound knowledge of, the producers, raw materials, and techniques. I saw him enjoy food without gluttony, thanks to his knowledge and his ability to taste.

Lastly, I would like to pay tribute to Folco Portinari, poet and writer (he was one of the editors of *La Gola*, the pioneering Italian magazine which revolutionized gastronomic discourse), with whom in the 1980s I formed, in the context of the Arcigola association,[13] a kind of intellectual partnership that still continues today. Though not without its disagreements, albeit always amicable and dictated by a sincere desire for an exchange of ideas, this relationship led, among other things, to the Slow Food Manifesto, which Portinari brilliantly wrote in 1986. His advice and criticism has always been most valuable, and he has taught me something more about the intellectual approach to gastronomy.

During the course of my life, since I began to travel widely, I have met other such figures all over the world. And while people from my own region were the first to influence me, among my later acquaintances of international standing I would like to mention another: Hugh Johnson, whom I consider to be the greatest connoisseur of wine and the greatest writer on the subject of the past century. *The Story of Wine*, his book on the history of wine, remains a classic work in its field. I was particularly impressed by his style, his methodological approach, and his ability to relate to farmers and wine producers all over the world. It was that style that made it possible for me to begin with wine and then continue the development which led to the ideas contained in this book.

This Diary, as the reader will have noticed, is primarily intended as a tribute to the people who have in some way or other changed my life, but I hope it will also help to emphasize how important personal education is for gastronomes and how alert one must be to discern in other people, by associating with them, those complex skills and different sensibilities that are the very essence of a gastronome, of the practice of this science that is so fascinating and yet (though hopefully not for much longer) so elusive.

1. GASTRONOMY

"Tell me what you eat and I'll tell you who you are," and "You are what you eat." The apparent obviousness of these two celebrated sayings by Jean-Anthelme Brillat-Savarin and Ludwig Feuerbach masks the infinite complexity which has to be taken into account if one is to demonstrate their truth; yet, at the same time, it asserts the absolute centrality of the role of food (a centrality which perhaps has been lost) if one wishes to inter-pret—and perhaps influence—the dynamics that underlie our society and our world.

Food is the primary defining factor of human identity, because what we eat is always a cultural product. If we accept the existence of a conceptual juxtaposition between nature and culture (between what is natural and what is artificial), food is the result of a series of processes (cultural ones, because they introduce artificial elements into the naturalness of things) that transform it from a completely natural base (the raw material) into the product of a culture (what we eat).

Man gathers, cultivates, domesticates, exploits, transforms, and reinterprets nature every time he eats. When he produces, he alters natural processes, influencing them in order to create his own food: the transition from a gathering economy to an agricultural one is the history of man as he settles, grows crops, raises livestock, and manipulates nature in response to his own needs. Then, when he goes on to prepare his meals, unlike other animals he uses more or less sophisticated technologies that transform the raw material: fire, fermentation, preserving, cook-ing. Lastly, when he consumes, he chooses more or less carefully how, what, where, and how much to eat.

All these processes, viewed in a historical perspective, indi-cate a titanic complexity, a human identity that is extremely unstable and constantly being redefined under the influence of exchanges, encounters, innovations, amalgamations, alliances, and conflicts. In order to convey the extent of that complexity, Massimo Montanari uses what seems to me a very apt metaphor for our identity, that of roots. The term "roots" is often used in a tendentious and mistaken way to evoke fixity, to underline and justify differences between peoples or, worse, between "races":

> The search for our roots never succeeds in identifying a point from which we started out, but only a twine of threads which grows thicker and more complicated the further back in time one goes. In this intricate system of additions and relations, it is not the roots but we ourselves who are the fixed point:

identity does not exist at the beginning but at the end of the process. If we must talk of roots, let us develop the metaphor and describe the history of our food culture as a plant that spreads out more widely the deeper it goes into the soil . . . The product is on the surface, visible, clear, well-defined: that is us. The roots are below the surface, abundant, numerous, wide-spreading: that is the history that has constructed us.[14]

I, too, would like to use this metaphor, and perhaps add a further meaning to it, because it will be a good way of restoring due importance to the food we eat and seeing what that food represents in the right proportions. Under the frenetic impulse of technocratic and reductionist thought, we have fallen into the temptation of neglecting the totality of the processes and inter-relations that enable us to eat every day, considering only the result, the food that we swallow. Yet these "roots" are crucial and must become a major subject of discussion again. To adapt Montanari, I would say that the product is on the surface, visible: that is what we have on our plate every day and what is most talked about. The roots are below—abundant, numerous, wide-spreading: they represent the way the food on our plate became food, the way it was created.

Food is the product of a region and of what has happened to it, of the people who live there, of its history, and of the relations it has established with other regions. One can talk about any place in the world simply by talking about the food that is produced and consumed there. In telling stories about food, one tells stories about agriculture, about restaurants, about trade, about local and global economies, about tastes, and even about famine. The peppers of Costigliole d'Asti are a symbol of globalization; amaranth and the wild herbs used in the Tehuacán soup tell of forgotten gastronomic knowledge and of ruined agricultural economies; the prawns of the Indian coasts are a manifestation of a mistaken concept of "development"; the vegetables in the farmers' market in San Francisco evoke the contradictions that well-meaning impulses can generate when they are grafted onto a system which is in itself somewhat perverse; (see Diaries

1, 2, 9, and 10, respectively). When one comes into contact with these stories, one understands more and more clearly that food is the primary means of interpreting reality, the world around us. Food reflects the complexity of the present-day world and of past history, the intertwining of cultures, and the overlapping of different philosophies of production.

The study of this amorphous mass of input and output, which is bordering on the chaotic, requires today a science that will examine it organically and take into account the multidisciplinarity that it necessarily involves—a science that will give new dignity and new tools to those who wish to study these subjects, and that, if I may be a trifle provocative, will be comprehensible even to those who insist on translating into figures things that are not calculable. A little humility, a more open-minded intellectual approach, and the recovery of a kind of knowledge that seems to have lost any "scientific" status may be a beginning.

1.1 Gastronomic science

There is a science that studies food, or rather the culture of food in every sense: *gastronomy*.

The word "gastronomy" is of Greek origin and is documented only sporadically in the major European languages before it was used in the title of a French poem by Joseph de Berchoux, *La Gastronomie, ou l'homme des champs à table*, which was printed in Paris in 1801 and translated into English in 1810. Note that the French title mentions the "man of the fields at table," thus in a sense connecting the farming world with the world of food consumption. But we will return to this subject later. For the moment, it is sufficient to observe that it was at the beginning of the nineteenth century that gastronomy began to achieve definition, and that the primary impulse came from French culture. After the French Revolution, a positive relationship was established between gastronomes and chefs, which helped to define and defend French cuisine over the next two centuries. During those years, modern catering was developing very fast in Paris: in 1804, there were five times as many restaurants as there had been in the prerevolutionary period; the number had risen to a thousand by 1825 and more than two thousand by 1834. Gastronomes made the fortunes and reputations of the chefs with their guides and their first critical writings. Gastronomic literature was born; among the most important authors were Jean-Anthelme Brillat-Savarin and Alexandre-Balthazar-Laurent Grimod de La Reynière, the true founders of modern gastronomy. The chefs themselves consolidated their popularity through the writings of Antoine Beauvilliers, Charles Durand, and Antonin Carême.

Etymologically, gastronomy means "the law of the stomach," or the set of rules that must be followed if one is to choose and consume food to the satisfaction of the stomach. Later definitions are only partial, because they define it as the "art of preparing and cooking food." When the word made its first official entry into the dictionary of the Académie Française in 1835, gastronomes were still defined as "hosts who choose, arrange, and offer a lavishly laid table."

In fact, the term can be extended beyond mere good eating and "living handsomely." The *choice* of foods, which seems to be the common denominator of all the main definitions, implies a rather wide range of knowledge, which touches on many other disciplines, both technological and humanistic. As we have seen, man has always altered nature in order to obtain the food he needs by means of various cultural processes, and the history of those processes is of daunting complexity to anyone who attempts to analyze them. To reduce gastronomy to "eating well" is a twofold error: first, because this definition implicitly accepts the common belief that the history of nutrition—economy and subsistence—and the history of gastronomy—culture and pleasure—are distinct subjects;[15] and secondly, because it only covers a small, and perhaps the least noble, part of the complex system of "roots" which underlie our food.

1.2 *The elite and hunger*

From the beginning, gastronomy had a markedly elitist connotation: after all, it was the dominant classes who wrote, for themselves, the recipe books and the first works of gastronomic criticism. It was therefore inevitable that gastronomy should be a science exclusively reserved for them. The "subordinate" culture of the poor and the rural population left no written records, and one can only guess from the recipe books of the aristocrats that the knowledge of the poor was expropriated by the ruling classes along with the right to pleasure. And yet the principal inventions in the history of gastronomy were made in the lower levels of society to respond to urgent needs: the absence of food, the perishability of produce, the need to transport or preserve it and therefore to minimize the impact of space and time on what we eat.

In 1801, when the word "gastronomy" appeared in the first writings on the subject, the main "law of the stomach" for most of the urban and rural population was still hunger, as it had been in earlier centuries. Only the abundance on the tables of the rich therefore had gastronomic dignity: it was thought—or at least said—that the methods of seasoning and cooking only concerned those who had no difficulty in obtaining adequate provisions. The poor and the hungry were from the outset denied all gastronomic dignity, though the gastronomic knowledge that they had built up and refined over centuries of adaptation to their land continued to be plundered and expropriated from them.

This fictitious separation between subsistence and pleasure may be said to have survived to this day. But in the meantime, starting in the years following World War II, the context has significantly changed. The great majority of the population of the Western world has solved the problem of obtaining provisions and its effect on the family budget. Although the figure of the gastronome is a product of the first post–French Revolutionary bourgeoisie, it has always reflected a tradition of noble, very rich cuisine, which has its roots in the recipe books of the royal courts. Gastronomy concerned the wealthy classes, who viewed the appetite and its satisfaction from countless different points of view, whetting it with taste, measuring it with pride.

The true bourgeois sense of gastronomy is far more modern, and it immediately begins to crumble when class differences lessen and food is no longer a means of asserting them. From 1950 onward, the term concerns larger sections of the population and the problem of *how* to choose food acquires other connotations; elitist gastronomy goes into crisis. It is no longer necessarily the well-to-do citizen who has the best diet, since he, too, buys poor-quality industrial products in soul-destroying supermarkets. In fact, unconscious and involuntary gastronomes spring up among those who live in contact with the land. Products that occur naturally or derive from the increasingly rare traditional forms of agriculture become delicacies for those who cannot easily obtain them.

Gastronomy is increasingly confined to the sphere of folklore and of play, not without coarse allusions to Pantagruelian abundance, which is in fact simply a way of exorcising our memory of hunger. The content of the current multitude of newspaper columns and color supplements, TV programs and game shows all devoted to the subject of food and gastronomy is the clearest proof of this development, which has taken on the dimensions of a social trend. There is no in-depth cultural analysis, no real knowledge of the subjects discussed: traditions add "color," and often pure nonsense is talked for the sake of audience figures. Try an experiment yourself: ask ten people to tell you what gastronomy is. They will talk vaguely of "good food"; they will mention the elitist connotations; some will tell you about shops that sell ready-made dishes, others will refer to the world of restaurants, chefs, and cookbooks enclosed with the daily newspapers. Nobody will say it's a science, and if you tell them it is, they'll probably think you're joking.

1.3 Pure folklore?

The histories of food, on the one hand, and of gastronomy on the other are separate and very different. The first represents economics and subsistence, serious subjects with a scientific basis; the second is associated with pleasure and the culture of food—

mere divertissement and hedonism, play and gluttony, of no importance at all. This fictitious separation has for centuries relegated gastronomy to the realm of folklore, denying it any scientific dignity and associating it only with the sphere of leisure, with the village fête, and with the media rage for regional and traditional products, with disputes about the ranking of restaurants.

If this situation has been taken to its most foolish extremes by the "popularization" of gastronomy that has been going on since World War II, the seeds of its scientific depreciation could already be seen in the writings of its founding fathers. Not even the traditional, elitist, almost "aristocratic" sense of the word has contributed to its "ennoblement." People who concern themselves with gastronomy, and therefore with pleasure, have always had to face the prejudice that pleasure is a sin (the religious influence on prevailing ideas), or at any rate not a serious matter. Just think of the well-known saying, "business before pleasure."

Even Brillat-Savarin, who wrote the fundamental *Physiologie du goût* (Physiology of Taste) in 1825, a year before his death and at the height of the French fashion for gastronomy, deep down was almost ashamed of it, or pretended to be. He published the book at his own expense, and his name was not even mentioned in the first edition. His real, or feigned, sense of "shame" is well expressed in the introductory "Dialogue Between the Author and His Friend":

> AUTHOR: . . . nevertheless I will not publish my book.
> FRIEND: Why not?
> AUTHOR: Because having dedicated myself by profession to serious studies, I fear that those who knew my book only by its title would think that I occupied myself with trifles.[16]

The author, a magistrate of thirty years' public service who had published weighty tomes in the fields of law and political economics (and also chemistry, in his youth), did not want to present an image of himself that was inconsistent with the status that he had achieved. Nevertheless, as he states in his preface, he was fairly sure of the importance of the arguments contained in his *Physiologie*:

> Considering the pleasure of the table in all its aspects, I had noticed some time ago that on this subject one could produce something better than cookbooks and that there was much to say about functions which are so important and so constant, and which have such a direct influence on happiness and even on business.[17]

His solution was to adopt the rhetorical device described by Jean-François Revel in his introduction to the work: "It was the charm of the composite composition to conceal the banal beneath the severe or the serious beneath the comical, the systematic in the unsystematic—the art of the cryptogram, which used to be one of the forms of discretion in literature but which today is no longer understood."[18]

I dwell at some length on Brillat-Savarin's work because it is an important landmark in the birth of modern gastronomy. As I have already mentioned, he and Grimod de La Reynière, in the successive issues of the *Almanach des Gourmands*, laid the foundations of modern gastronomic literature and introduced elements of modern gastronomic criticism. I am aware of both the limitations and brilliance of *Physiologie du goût*, and I do not wish to compete with the historians of gastronomy; as a matter of fact, Brillat-Savarin did not invent anything, and a historical account would require deeper analysis than can be given in these few lines. But *Physiologie*, though its style is playful and only half-serious, defines clearly and skillfully all the basic elements that we ourselves need today to found a new gastronomic science (the book is also a significant achievement as a literary exercise, for, apart from the recipe books, this was a genre that had no particularly distinguished models at the time). If the subject has until now been confined to the realms of folklore, it is partly due to Brillat-Savarin, undoubtedly; but if we read his *Physiologie* with a slightly more scientific approach, we find a definition of gastronomy that I would like to take as the basis for the modest arguments presented in this book:

> Gastronomy is the reasoned knowledge of everything concerning man insofar as he eats . . . It is gastronomy that moves the growers, the winemakers, the fishermen, and the numerous family of cooks, whatever the title or qualification under which they mask their concern with the preparation of food. Gastronomy belongs to natural history, because of the classification it makes of kinds of food; to physics, because of the various tests and analyses to which it subjects that food; to cooking, because of its concern with the art of preparing food and making it pleasant to the taste; to trade, because of its search for the means of buying at the best possible price that which it consumes and of selling at the highest possible profit that which it puts on sale; to political economics, because of the resources it provides for the financial authorities and the methods of exchange that it establishes between the nations.[19]

Here, in the third "Meditation" of the treatise, we already find all the complex elements of gastronomy as a multidisciplinary science, in a description that takes account of the agricultural, economic, scientific, technical, social, and cultural processes that are involved in nutrition. Much of the work's originality lies in this definition, which claims due dignity for gastronomy, in a vision characterized by good sense and a surprisingly modern ability to grasp the complexity of things.

Embracing this multidisciplinarity, then, *in toto* and without reservation, though fully aware of my own limitations, I would like to begin from this point, from Brillat-Savarin's definition, endorsing both its first sentence and its structure, opening the mind to chaos, but rejecting the "folkloristic" approach, though not spurning the element of playfulness, much less that of pleasure. This is, rather, a vision which regards play and pleasure as serious matters, which draws on disciplines old and new in the light of developments during the two centuries that have passed since the publication of *Physiologie du goût*, and which implies important reflections—to return to that other favorite aphorism of Brillat-Savarin—on who we are, that is, on what we eat.

Many great friendships arise by chance among the tables of restaurants, during convivial encounters that happen to reveal elective affinities between gastronomes; these affinities are then cemented by time, leading to fruitful collaborations, fertile exchanges of ideas, and fascinating human adventures. So it was with Alice Waters. She was, at the time, the one person in the United States who embraced from the outset the embryonic ideas of Slow Food that I was then trying to propagate. I met her during my first visit to California, in February 1988, having made a particular point of visiting her restaurant Chez Panisse, which everyone seemed to agree was the best in the San Francisco area. Her fame had spread all over the United States because, apart from her wonderful cuisine, Waters had reawoken the native pride of the young Californian gastronomic culture (and by extension that of the whole United States), along with a profound feeling of respect for the environment and for the traditional knowledge of that land.

The cuisine that she purveyed at Chez Panisse was strongly influenced by her experiences in France and Italy, but equally closely linked to local farming and to the wealth of knowledge that the numerous immigrant families in this part of the States had brought with them and handed on. The exceptional quality of her dishes has defined a very personal style, which has always made the organoleptic characteristics of the raw materials its main ingredient—something very unusual in the homeland of industrialized agriculture and fast food.

Waters was educated in that fertile world of alternative culture that centered around Berkeley in the late 1960s, a movement which among other things asserted the reestablishment of a peaceful and harmonious relationship with nature. As a result, from the start her restaurant was a rallying point for the nascent environmentalist culture. Amost from its beginning Chez Panisse has used only raw materials deriving from organic agriculture and local farms. Waters may truly be described as the leading inspiration of the organic movement in the United States: she and a few friends began to promote the cause of cleaner agriculture in the 1970s, and their success can be seen today in the great care taken with sustainability and in the quantities of organic crops now produced in California.

I can vouch for the fact that eating at Waters's restaurant is a remarkable gastronomic experience. It is astonishing for the delicacy and care with which her chefs cook, but even more so for the clarity of the flavors: they manage to bring out the taste of the vegetables in a way that I have rarely encountered anywhere else in the world. The mix between a refined culinary technique and a choice of produce that is positively manic in its respect for correctness in the production process and for the geographical proximity of suppliers guarantees wonderful results. Even the unassuming flavor of French beans as an accompaniment to one of the dishes seems almost like a miracle of nature, something absolutely amazing.

But Waters is not just a brilliant cook and a paladin of sustainable agriculture: over the years, I have seen another side of the original approach she has been determined to pursue in her gastronomic venture. In 2000—I always drop by whenever I'm in San Francisco—she took me to see a project she had recently initiated: "The Edible Schoolyard." The Martin Luther King Jr. Middle School in Berkeley has almost a thousand students; many of them are Latino or African-American, and it cannot exactly be described as an elite school. But these children, at least as far as their school is concerned, are lucky. Waters has created at their school something I still consider to be the true masterpiece of her gastronomic career. It is what is usually called a school garden—a kitchen garden tended by the children, who thus assimilate the basics of agriculture, but above all learn to recognize the vegetables, their characteristics, and their qualities. The originality of the project lies in the fact that the children not only have the chance to grow their own food in an urban context, where eating habits have completely eradicated every kind of gastronomic education, but they also learn the rudiments of cooking, because they are taught how to process what they cultivate. Hence the name, the Edible Schoolyard.

It is an undeniable fact that the poorest children and teenagers in the big American cities no longer eat at home; their parents do not cook at all, and the family does not come together for meals. Food is bought either in the form of prepared meals from the supermarket or at the local fast-food restaurant. The obliteration of gastronomic knowledge in the United States has been total, and its effects on public health are rapidly making themselves felt. The Edible Schoolyard is a way of teaching these children to cook, to recognize the best kinds of food; it is a way of refining their sense of taste and their sensibility. It is a model that ought to be imitated all over the world; all schools should devote particular attention to gastronomic themes, and they should not wait to do so until the very last moment, when the situation is almost beyond repair, as it is in the suburbs of the American cities.

In this respect Waters has opened my eyes: she has found a formula that works, a playful and entertaining way of teaching gastronomy to children and at the same time feeding them a healthy school lunch. It is no coincidence that she is now the international vice-president of Slow Food; her career as a chef is a living example of an approach that transcends the canonical forms of the cook's profession, that goes beyond the mere practicalities of running a restaurant, and that crosses all the borders of gastronomic multidisciplinarity. She is a crucial figure, who has absorbed all the complexity of being a gastronome into her everyday life, becoming the creator of a new way of operating in the world of food, in the very nation responsible for some of the worst aberrations ever seen in nutritional history, with enormous repercussions on the whole planet.

....

{DIARY 6} THE FLORENCE GROUP
....

On February 4–5, 2003, I attended the first meeting of the Commission on the Future of Food, a working group set up on the initiative of the Regional Council of Tuscany.[20] My particular task was to draw up a *Manifesto on the Future of Food,* to be presented at subsequent meetings of the World Trade Organization (WTO). This was the first time I had ever received an official invitation to make a contribution as an eco-gastronome and to exchange ideas with leading scholars, antiglobalization activists, and ecologists from all over the world. The organizers' aim—which proved successful—was that this first meeting should be an opportunity for people to get to know one another and begin discussing the strategies that need to be adopted in order to bring about a worldwide revival of "food sovereignty"—that is to say, of people's right to choose what kind of agriculture they practice, how they eat, and how much they eat, in accordance with their economic potential and the traditional knowledge they possess.

My first impressions of the meeting were very striking: gathered in a sumptuous room of the palace that houses the Regional Council of Tuscany, in Via Cavour, Florence, you felt isolated from the world. The magnificence of the room was slightly off-putting; at least, it created a sense of solemnity that was perhaps excessive, even given the seriousness of the meeting. The other members of the group seemed to know each other very well; they were, after all, part of the elite of world activism, and they had already met and worked together several times before. I knew only two of them well, because until then my movement had kept slightly apart from purely antiglobalization dynamics and from the "official" ecological groups. We had always preferred to work directly in the field, through selective and very concrete projects such as the Presidia—small-scale projects devoted to the preservation of a specific food product (see especially pp. 162–64)—while our "ecological consciences" as gastronomes were in fact very young: a degree of healthy respect and the belief that it was better to concentrate on real activities than on words had induced us to remain independent.

The fact that most of those present had never had any personal contact with me or my movement probably generated a certain amount of suspicion, accompanied by the usual stereotype of the Italian gastronome: an affable fellow, very fond of his food, somewhat hedonistic, and a great expert on the culinary marvels of his country. That a fantastic buffet had been prepared on the floor below, using products saved and protected by Slow Food, must have reinforced this prejudice.

The meeting opened to the apocalyptic tones of Edward Goldsmith, who took everyone aback with his forecast that life on Earth would come to an end within a few decades. The manner in which the founder of the magazine *The Ecologist* began his speech may have been a little rhetorical, but considering the situation in which our planet finds itself today, perhaps he was not too far from the truth. At any rate, this speech was followed by a series of typically ecologist criticisms and denunciations; the main focus of attack as far as the future of food was concerned was the damage caused by industrial systems of agriculture and the iniquities of international trade.

I listened with interest, but I was also impatient for them to start talking about food. Not that what they said was not relevant to the subject—I know it is important to analyze the systems of production that are used around the world, to question their quality, verify their sustainability, and ensure that all other cultures and societies of the world are respected, but if people do not take into account the "gastronomic" side of things, they make the same mistake, in reverse, as gastronomes make when they talk about food without knowing where it comes from, confining themselves to learned disquisitions on taste. In other words, I felt the lack of an all-embracing vision of reality, and it seemed to me that people were making more or less the same mistake as the reductionists and the overspecialists. To put it plainly: a gastronome who has no environmental sensibility is a fool; but an ecologist who has no gastronomic sensibility is a sad figure, unable to understand the cultures in which he wants to work. What we need, then, is eco-gastronomy.

So my speech caught the meeting somewhat off guard. Logic would have demanded that I discuss Slow Food's ecological vision, using the same language as the others and perhaps singing the praises of our concrete efforts to preserve biodiversity. I certainly did not neglect to inform the others about our projects, but my whole speech centered on the right to pleasure, and especially on gastronomy. My basic argument was as follows: pleasure is a human right because it is physiological; we cannot fail to feel pleasure when we eat. Anyone who eats the food that is available to him, devising the best ways of making it agreeable, feels pleasure.

The traditional cultures have created a vast heritage of recipes, ways of preparing and processing local or easily accessible food. This is true even of those areas in the world that are most seriously affected by the problems of malnutrition today; just think of the gastronomic culture of India. These forms of knowledge are intimately linked with biodiversity and show us both a way of using it and a way of defending it. Moreover, they give pleasure: organoleptic pleasure of course, but also intellectual pleasure, as one might call it, because they are the symbol of a particular culture.

To reject pleasure in the belief that it only accompanies abundance is a serious strategic mistake. Even the Food and Agriculture Organization, which has always regarded pleasure as a secondary consideration compared with the serious emergencies it has to solve, is currently reviewing its attitude. We should not give food aid without first considering the context of the countries that are in difficulty; we should not try to stimulate agricultural development by introducing elements that are external in origin or completely alien to the local ecosystem. Any such attempt at intervention is bound to fail, and may well cause even more serious damage.

When the group heard me mention pleasure, I saw the expressions on their faces—and my impression was confirmed by a colleague of mine who was present at the meeting: their preconceived notion of the hedonistic glutton had been satisfied. But this was only their first reaction, because fortunately they were highly intelligent and open-minded people. After the initial response, perhaps of slight amusement, there was a vigorous discussion on the subject, notable for a speech by Vandana Shiva, who spoke about the importance of gastronomy for the defense of traditional kinds of vegetables (it was on this occasion that I struck up a close friendship and collaboration with Shiva, who is the founder and director of the Research Foundation for Science, Technology, and Ecology in India and an important activist for biodiversity). Her argument was that there was no point in persuading small farmers to preserve or reintroduce the seeds of their traditional plants if you did not also teach them how to use and cook them. Even Goldsmith, giving one of his infectious smiles and using the same flowery language with which he had foretold the apocalypse, agreed with me, admitting that he had never thought about the problem before. The result was that in the *Manifesto on the Future of Food*, which was drawn up after several other meetings of this kind and presented at a meeting held in July 2003 in San Rossore, Tuscany, the introduction ended with these words:

> The entire conversion from local small-scale food production for local communities, to large-scale export-oriented monocultural production has also brought the melancholy decline of the traditions, cultures, and cooperative pleasures and convivialities associated for centuries with community-based production and markets, thereby diminishing the experience of direct food-growing, and the long celebrated joys of sharing food grown by local hands from local lands. [See Appendix p. 259, for full text.]

I considered it a minor victory that the text included a defense of the right to pleasure, and although it was not easy, after the others' initial doubts about my position we all developed a sense of solidarity in the writing of a document which I think has yet to be given the attention it deserves by the powerful of our planet. The members of the group, in their several fields and each through their own activities, are carrying on the work, more convinced than ever that it is time to create alternatives if we are to change, and save, the future of food. And gastronomes like me are part of the project.

In the autumn of 2001, I developed liver problems which led to my spending several periods in the hospital. The treatment was long and tedious, though happily effective, and it gave me firsthand experience of what had long been a personal conviction of mine. This unpleasant illness became an experience that, seen through the eyes of a gastronome, revealed all the profundity and complexity of our relationship with culinary pleasure, which is usually considered unhealthy and conducive to disease. The fact that I have been compelled since my illness to follow a more spartan diet, and abstain from drinking alcohol, has taught me to refine my relationship with food. I have become more sensitive, and I learned that I can use all the knowledge I acquired in the gustatory-olfactory field from wine-tasting and apply it to other products. For example, I have discovered the variety and complexity of the smells and tastes of tea (a whole new world has opened up before me); I have concentrated on the differences between the various varieties of fruit and vegetables; and I have become more aware of the types of wheat and of the kind of treatment they have been subjected to before being turned into pasta or bread.

In short, my senses have become even more acute and able to perceive nuances. I have left behind me that period of my life when I enjoyed food perhaps to an excessive extent, sometimes losing sight of the real meaning of tasting, and in effect proving right those people who regard pleasure as the antagonist of health. What I have come to understand is that this antagonism does not exist; it is all a question of training and moderation, of a sense of restraint. Some might ask why it was necessary for me to fall ill in order to understand this. My reply is that no experience is without its usefulness, and that even my contact with hospital food taught me a gastronomic lesson. I began to attempt critical assessments of these collective kitchens; I wrote rigorous reviews of them (and was by no means too hard on them), using the same criteria as I used for restaurants, and I found further confirmation of the fact that our relationship with food must be moderate, certainly, but should never be mortifying. It is not clear why all over the world in "enforced residences"—prisons, hospitals, and other such places—food should always be a secondary consideration, pure sustenance devoid of taste and gastronomic interest, unconnected with the locality, the season (and therefore lacking all freshness), or any kind of naturalness.

That experience convinced me that good food can in fact be a very useful therapeutic aid, a way of alleviating and making more bearable all kinds of suffering, whether physical or mental. I began to urge my doctors to explore this link between pleasure and health, which had never been scientifically studied even by nutritionists, let alone by medical professionals; I found among them some very intelligent people who responded to my provocations in a constructive manner.

Food has always had a medical connotation in all cultures, even the most primitive; but somehow all this has degenerated so that modern science is largely nutritionist in its approach, subdividing foods according to their nutritional characteristics—with no thought given to the taste of a dish or to its beneficial effects considered as an integral whole, including both the nutritional and the pleasurable aspects. A gastronome, then, must have medical concerns, but hopefully doctors, too, will begin to develop a gastronomic sensibility. I am sure that this would lead to new and interesting treatments and diets, achieving results that would seem almost miraculous even to a scientist.

2. THE NEW GASTRONOMY: A DEFINITION

Gastronomy is the reasoned knowledge of everything that concerns man as he eats; it facilitates choice, because it helps us to understand what quality is.

Gastronomy enables us to experience educated pleasure and to learn pleasurably. Man as he eats is culture; thus gastronomy is culture, both material and immaterial.

Choice is a human right; gastronomy is freedom of choice. Pleasure is also everybody's right and as such must be as responsible as possible; gastronomy is a creative matter, not a destructive one. Knowledge is everybody's right as well, but also a duty, and gastronomy is education.

Gastronomy is part of the following fields:

- *botany*, *genetics*, and the other *natural sciences*, in its classification of the various kinds of food, thus making possible their conservation;

- *physics* and *chemistry*, in its selection of the best products and its study of how they are processed;

- *agriculture*, *zootechnics*, and *agronomy*, in its concern with the production of good and varied raw materials;

- *ecology*, because man, in producing, distributing, and consuming food, interferes with nature and transforms it to his advantage;

- *anthropology*, because it contributes to the study of the history of man and his cultural identities;

- *sociology*, from which it takes its methods of analyzing human social behavior;

- *geopolitics*, because peoples form alliances and come into conflict partly, indeed chiefly, over the right to exploit the earth's resources;

- *political economics*, because of the resources it provides, and because of the methods of exchange that it establishes between nations;

- *trade*, because of its search for the means of buying at the best possible price that which it consumes and of selling at the highest possible profit that which it puts on sale;

- *technology*, *industry*, and the *know-how* of people, in its search for new methods of processing and preserving food inexpensively;

- *cooking*, in its concern with the art of preparing food and making it pleasing to the taste;

- *physiology*, in its ability to develop the sensorial capacities that enable us to recognize what is good;

- *medicine*, in its study of the healthiest way of eating;

- *epistemology*, because, through a necessary reconsideration of the scientific method and of the criteria of knowledge that enable us to analyze the path food travels from the field to the table, and vice versa, it helps us to interpret the reality of our complex, globalized world; it helps us to choose.

Gastronomy enables us to live the best life possible using the resources available to us and stimulates us to improve our existence.

Gastronomy is a science that analyzes happiness. Through food, which is a universal and immediate language, a component of identity, and an object of exchange, it reveals itself as one of the most powerful forms of peace diplomacy.

2.1 On botany, the natural sciences, and genetics,
or On biodiversity and its seeds

Anyone who has the good fortune to view Bartolomeo Bimbi's huge canvases depicting Cosimo de' Medici's sumptuous Renaissance botanic gardens or some of the rare illustrations from one of the only 170 surviving copies of Giorgio Gallesio's monumental work, *Pomona Italiana*, will see in those paintings and drawings traces of a biodiversity that is now lost and forgotten.

Gallesio was born in Finale Ligure in 1772 and died in Florence in 1839. He was a man of many hats: farmer, magistrate, deputy, public official, and diplomat. He is chiefly remembered, however, for his enlightened contribution to the science that studies the vegetable kingdom, and in particular for introducing to Italy that branch of botany, pomology (the science of fruit-growing), which was already widespread in other parts of Europe.

Pomona Italiana was an ambitious and unprecedented publishing project: for twenty-five years, Gallesio traveled the length of the Italian peninsula from north to south, recording, describing, and classifying the principal existing varieties of fruit. The results were published in forty-one fascicules containing more than 160 color plates of extraordinary beauty and meticulously accurate reproduction.[21]

Through its illustrations and text, *Pomona Italiana* gives us a picture of the heritage of Italian fruit in the early nineteenth century. The value of this work to scientific research is immense, especially for scholars working on the conservation and improvement of genetic resources in fruit-growing. It is an important contribution to our knowledge of Italian biodiversity, in that it describes the history of many varieties and can help us understand what has been lost and how easily such losses can occur.

In our own time, too, the problem of cataloguing the varieties of fruit and vegetables is a very topical, indeed rather urgent, one. The strong impulse toward high productivity in agriculture on a largely industrial basis has led to a rapid selection—not only by natural means, but also through hybridization and even through "creation" using genetically modified organisms (GMOs)—of new vegetable and animal varieties that suit the new production processes of our era. The square peppers of Asti and many varieties of Latin American corn, for example, have had to give way to hybrids, or at any rate to more productive varieties. The Millennium Ecosystem Assessment report gives an account of the massive reduction in biodiversity that has already taken place on our planet and which continues with increasing speed. Among the main causes indicated in the report are modern farming methods.

The *Fatal Harvest*[22] collection of studies gives some data on the loss in biodiversity in the United States alone: 80.6 percent of the varieties of tomato became extinct between 1903 and 1983, as did 92.8 percent of the varieties of lettuce, 86.2 percent of the varieties of apple and, during the same period, 90.8 percent of the varieties of field corn and 96.1 percent of the varieties of sweet corn. Of the over five thousand existing varieties of potato, only four form the vast majority of those cultivated for commercial purposes in the United States; two types of pea account for 96 percent of American cultivations, and six types of corn for 71 percent of the total.

The seed multinationals seek to impose their seeds on the market by every means possible. Natural selection, which farmers traditionally carried out after each harvest by putting aside the seeds of the plants that had the best characteristics, is scarcely practiced any longer, except in areas where people still use what are regarded as "old-fashioned" agricultural methods. Seeds are now bought year by year from the firms that have developed the varieties that give a more abundant harvest: the objectives are quantity at all costs and resistance to the herbicides, which are often produced by the seed industries themselves. And now we have GMOs, the culmination of this "unnatural" evolution. Twelve thousand years of gradual selection made by the farmers have been wiped out in a mere fifty years in the pursuit of commercial targets.

This trade in seeds gives rise to absurd situations all over the world. In Saskatchewan, Canada, for example, the farmer Percy Schmeiser has been engaged for the past ten years in a long and exhausting legal battle against the multinational Monsanto, which accused him of illegally taking some of their genetically modified seeds. He was charged with violating the patent that the American multinational holds on a particular kind of transgenic rape, but he has always maintained that his field was contaminated by his neighbor's crops.[23]

This is only one of the many examples that could be mentioned. Another is occurring even now in the region of Karnataka in India, where more than six hundred farmers a year commit suicide (in India as a whole the number of cases runs into thousands) because they are unable to pay the debts they incur in order to buy seeds and the chemicals that are needed to make them grow. Or take the case of Mexico, where even in the remotest areas—the very cradle of biodiversity as far as corn is concerned—the luxuriant, almost wild countryside is broken up and dotted with posters for either Coca-Cola or the seed multinationals that advertise "miraculous" varieties of corn (the fact that corn is *advertised* is in itself rather weird, in certain areas of Mexico).

The seed trade is evidently the one on which the multinationals of agroindustry have chosen to focus their attention in order to control the market. There can be no doubt that GMOs, even leaving aside all ethical, health-related, or ecological considerations, are the most underhanded and powerful weapon in a commercial strategy aiming to dominate the entire productive process, starting with the first principle of life itself: the seed.

The reduction in biodiversity thus has a strategic importance in the commercial plans of the multinationals, and it is not just biodiversity, or the raw materials, that are lost; along with them are lost the related knowledge, techniques, and economies. The loss goes much further than simple biology.

So the natural sciences and genetics are of great importance from a gastronomic point of view as well: the contributions they can make, through the creation of germplasm banks and the study and cataloguing of existing varieties, thus pointing research in a different direction from that of high productivity, are without doubt where the future of our food lies. Working in these fields in order to safeguard and improve the traditional varieties or the old agricultural genetic technologies (putting the best seeds aside and sowing them again each year) is a prime necessity. Since the private sector is unlikely to take on such a task, those who finance research from public funds will have to take the first step, by promoting joint research projects in collaboration with the farmers, trying out a new approach that encourages "official" science to work with the world of traditional knowledge. Projects of this kind have already been launched in France, with interesting results. It would be useful to study them carefully and, if possible, replicate them elsewhere, especially in areas where traditional knowledge is still deeply rooted and in serious danger of rapid extinction, as in the developing countries.

2.2 On physics and chemistry, or On techniques for creating flavor

The use of fire to cook food is an operation that distinguishes man from animals. Man, unlike the rest of the animal kingdom, cooks instead of merely taking what exists in nature. Fire (and by extension all the other ways of preparing food) is the first cultural step in the process that makes food itself a cultural factor.

But the effect of fire on raw materials is first and foremost a question of physics and chemistry. Material is processed in order to make it edible, preservable, transportable, and as pleasant as possible. Fire cooks, produces the smoke you need if you wish to smoke food, and makes sterilization possible by generating very high temperatures. The laws that govern these processes, after being unknown for centuries, were finally demonstrated simply through culinary empiricism, but progress in the scientific disciplines also led to new inventions.

With the onset of industrialization, the nutritional needs of those who worked in factories and therefore had little time for cooking changed (the working day was much longer then—and to think that today we complain about not having time to cook our meals!). At the same time, industrialization brought new developments in the food industry, which relies on chemistry for its ability to mass-produce food that is packaged and in most cases virtually ready for use. The combination of new needs and of new discoveries in the field of food technology made possible a great expansion of the food industry, but it later turned out that the use of chemistry had been too indiscriminate, resulting in food scandals, new diseases, and the impoverishment of our diet in nutritional value and taste.

The golden age of the application of chemistry to the food sector was the second half of the nineteenth century and the innovators included: Julius Maggi with his powdered soups and stock cubes; Justus von Liebig (the same man who invented chemical fertilizers) with his meat extract; Hippolyte Mège-Mouriès with margarine; Carl Knorr and more powdered soups; Rudolph Oeteker with his yeast; Wilhelm Haarmann, who invented vanillin; and Francesco Cirio in Italy, who began producing his preserves in a small workshop in Piazza della Repubblica, Turin (the spot is now marked by a poorly preserved plaque). The same period saw the invention of Coca-Cola, chewing gum, and canned pineapple. Whether or not these pioneers realized how revolutionary their inventions were, it was they who initiated the industrial production of food on a mass scale, which foreshadowed the later industrialization of agricultural techniques.

The present-day food industry needs no introduction—we all know it only too well. It churns out all kinds of comestibles; it even reproduces traditional dishes and carries individual food cultures around the world, at least in their more obvious manifestations. At the supermarket, you can buy frozen pizza, Mexican sauces, and the ingredients for burritos, precooked curry or paella to heat up in a saucepan, and soups and broths from all over the world. There are also invented products such as chocolate snacks, potato chips, and processed cheese slices. These creations have become the epitome of the industry itself; the trademarks on the brightly colored packets are more important than their contents, and the products inside bear little resemblance in aspect, smell, or taste to anything that occurs in nature.

What happened, although it originated as a response to a real social need of the families who worked in the factories (but soon proved an excellent way of making money, too), in fact completely subverted the rules of food processing. The treatments were so unnatural and so violent—dehydration, freeze-drying, deep-freezing, et cetera—that additional elements had to be invented just so that the raw materials could regain some semblance of naturalness and some distant echo of their original taste. Nothing in nature resembles the chicken nuggets that are served in fast-food restaurants. It is impossible to associate them with the fowl they come from; their shape is completely artificial, and the raw material does not taste remotely like chicken, partly because of the selection of meat (production offcuts and innards) from factory-farmed birds, and partly because of the processing it has undergone—a production line which minces, sterilizes, adds thickeners, emulsifiers, and stabilizers, and finally freezes it. This is where chemistry comes in, for it can "reconstruct" out of nothing—create a taste, a smell, a texture. The industry of "artificial and natural" flavorings and of the various additives that we find listed among the ingredients is flourishing but also elusive. One of the rare descriptions of it was given by Eric Schlosser in his *Fast Food Nation*:

> The IFF (International Flavors & Fragrances) plant in
> Dayton is a huge pale blue building with a modern office
> complex attached to the front... Wonderful smells drifted
> through the hallways... and hundreds of little glass bottles sat
> on laboratory tables and shelves... The long chemical names
> on the little white labels were as mystifying to me as medieval
> Latin. They were the odd-sounding names of things that
> would be mixed and poured and turned into new substances,
> like magic potions... IFF's snack and savory lab is responsible
> for the flavor of potato chips, corn chips, breads, crackers,
> breakfast cereals, and pet food. The confectionery lab devises
> the flavor for ice cream, cookies, candies, toothpastes, mouth-
> washes, and antacids... In addition to being the world's
> largest flavor company, IFF manufactures the smell of six of

the ten best-selling fine perfumes in the United States, including Estée Lauder's Beautiful, Clinique's Happy, Lancôme's Trésor, and Calvin Klein's Eternity... All of these aromas are made through the same basic process: the manipulation of volatile chemicals to create a particular smell.[24]

Man has succeeded in separating the flavor from the product, thus making it possible to recombine each at will. The industrial process of food production has no respect for the raw material and its original characteristics, for it is able to reproduce its consistency, appearance, and flavor in a laboratory. As a result, food labels become incomprehensible. The following are the ingredients that create an apricot flavor in ice cream, for example: heptyl acetate, santalyl acetate, phenylpropylic alcohol, amyl phenylacetate, phenylethyl dimethylcarbinol, benzyl formiate, geranyl isobutyrate, methyl isobutyrate, butyl propinate, and heptyl propinate.

These compounds are often concealed under the term "natural or artificial flavorings." The fact that some of these flavorings are described as "natural" does not mean that they really are. It only means that they are obtained from a natural substance. *How* they are extracted, by more or less sophisticated chemical processes that are not always beneficial to human health, does not matter: from a legal point of view they are "natural." As Schlosser notes: "Even though an almond flavor (benzaldehyde) is obtained from natural sources, such as peach and apricot kernels, it contains traces of hydrocyanic acid, a deadly poison."[25]

Today, research into the effects of flavorings and other chemical products has begun to light up what seemed a dark and impenetrable sky. Ingesting these products, even in microscopic quantities but continuously throughout our lives, exposes us to another form of pollution whose effects have yet to be fully investigated. There is talk of an increase in the number of allergies, and of poisonings, small or large though rarely fatal, by carcinogenic substances (such as that denominated Sudan 1, a chemical coloring agent sometimes used in food), which have been discovered after people have been unwittingly consuming them in large quantities for years. Certainly, there is a risk of these compounds dulling our sense of taste. They raise our threshold of perception to the point where we think natural products organoleptically poor, and they homogenize all flavors, depriving us of the joy of experiencing the natural diversity of taste, which is so rich, varied, and gratifying to the palate. At a cultural level, moreover, food additives have turned flavor into a marketing tool. Now there is actually such a thing as "food design," which constructs the flavor of a product and even the product itself, in accordance with the results of market research; it adapts an industrial process to meet the supposed demand and then selects the cheapest suitable raw material. In effect, it turns on its head the process whereby man, in order to feed himself, starts with what he finds in nature and tries to improve its flavor. Food design starts with the flavor it wants to obtain; all other considerations come later.

Chemistry and physics are part of modern gastronomic science because they can help us restore due prominence to taste, which is intimately linked to what is indisputably the central element, the raw material. They can help us organize industrial food production in a sustainable way and prevent the production of substances that are harmful to our health, unmasking those who abuse the concept of food design. They can explain what happens in the process that leads from the chicken to the nugget, for example: they can tell us what our food really contains, so that we can avoid the continuation of what, for more than a century, has been a deception practiced on consumers.

Just as these two sciences enabled man to perform the miracle of dissecting food and reassembling it at will, so they can help us restore its naturalness, its original flavor, to study the traditional techniques of preservation and processing, to accord them their rightful dignity and perhaps even improve them, bringing out all their potential. All this can be done without distorting the traditional methods for the sake of mass-producing large quantities, without stealing them from the original productive communities to patent them or trying to replicate them artificially, with all the risks that this involves.

If chemistry can place itself at the service of gastronomy—as it was in the past when food processing was performed in a scientifically more unconscious way and when empiricism indissolubly linked the preparation of food to its naturalness—it will benefit our health, our knowledge, and our enjoyment of flavor.

2.3 On agriculture and ecology,
or On the techniques for producing sustainable food

During the last fifty years, agriculture has become increasingly industrialized. The introduction of elements external to the natural system in which agriculture is practiced, such as pesticides and chemical fertilizers, has rapidly compromised the salubriousness of food and of the environment. The survey, at the beginning of this book, of the damage that man has done to the earth showed that it is mainly attributable to modern systems of food production. The reduction of biodiversity has reached unprecedented levels and continues unabated.

Brillat-Savarin included agriculture among the subjects that are part of gastronomy, but later, with the spread of industrial methods, the two disciplines were completely separated, widening the gaps between the different phases of harvesting, processing, and consumption. Having lost its connection to gastronomy, agriculture has maintained ties only with the industry of food production. So we have reached the absurd situation where there are children today who eat chicken nuggets but have never seen a live chicken and don't even know what one looks like. We have completely severed the link which until after World War II tied people to the earth with respect to food. Those who lived in the country, but also those who had moved to the cities not more than two generations earlier, had always been able to see where their food came from. Gastronomic knowledge was passed down almost automatically from generation to generation. Nowadays, that umbilical cord of ancient knowledge no longer exists, and more than ever before production and consumption seem like two completely distinct phases, which are both greatly the poorer for their total lack of mutual knowledge.

It is this lack of knowledge that leads many of us to eat, unthinkingly, in fast-food restaurants.

And yet common sense would suggest that a gastronome, or even someone who would not describe himself as such, should demand to know everything about what he eats: its provenance, the processes it has undergone, and the people who have been involved. An interest in agriculture, its evolution, and its changes should be a priority for everyone who eats: "Eating is an agricultural act," in the magisterial definition of Wendell Berry, the Kentucky farmer, poet, and essayist.[26] But for many people that is not the case, and as well as harming ourselves and paying for it in loss of flavor and poverty of diet, we automatically become accomplices of the devastation that is wrought on the earth by the spread of unsustainable agricultural methods.

The gastronome should know about agriculture, because he wants to know about his food and because he wants to support those agricultural methods that preserve biodiversity and the associated tastes and knowledge. It goes without saying, too, that given the state to which we have reduced the earth, the gastronome ought to have an environmental conscience and be well informed about ecology. I repeat: a gastronome who does not have an environmental conscience is a fool, because without it he will be deceived in every way possible and will allow the earth, from which he draws the essence of his work, to die. In the same way, it may be said that an ecologist who is not also something of a gastronome is a sad character, who besides not being able to enjoy nature and missing out on the pleasure of eating, is indirectly prepared to do serious damage to the ecosystem by the simple act of eating incorrectly.

I am putting agriculture and ecology together in a single discipline, because I think they are inseparable: anyone who tills the land and raises livestock works with nature and must not exploit and kill it. At the same time, environmentalists must understand that gastronomy is the art of producing food in harmony with the surrounding environment and that organic monocultures, for example, are not sustainable: even if you do not use chemical products, you can destroy the environment by eliminating biodiversity (such as woodland, other plants) in favor of a single variety that is produced in large quantities. The same happens if you introduce varieties that are foreign to the existing ecosystem; they may be organic, but they are alien to the environment and may cause serious damage to it. Above all, those who cultivate the land must not forget taste. If a product is not good, there is no point in it being organic; if it is not good and is alien to the local culture, it may be useful in responding to an emergency, but it will not permanently solve the problem of hunger or of certain kinds of pollution.

Agriculture and ecology must be a single entity, then, and both combine in gastronomy, the only sustainable way to produce food. Together they form a discipline so wide-ranging as to be capable of controlling and harmonizing the complexity that characterizes the food system. In fact, we are talking of a science which already exists—which has been described as, and I think really is, the true way toward a sustainable future: agroecology.

Agroecology is a young science that already boasts several different schools, all of which are, broadly speaking, based on the assumption that ecosystems, just as they are, possess all the means they need to regulate themselves. In order to grow crops and raise livestock, we must manipulate the environment gently, with due respect to local biodiversity, traditional culture, and the rhythms of nature. Miguel Altieri, professor of agroecology at the University of Berkeley in California, gives a good definition of the subject in the course of an interview:

> For my school, agroecology is a science which is highly influenced by traditional agricultural science. We recognize this traditional knowledge as a science which has the same dignity as all the other sciences. Agroecology seeks a common matrix of dialogue between different realms, between this traditional knowledge and Western science, putting them on the same level. It is not a question of proving the validity of traditional knowledge by scientific methods, but of connecting the different notions for use in particular cases.

For example, in many parts of the world traditional farmers classify the soil by putting it in their mouths and tasting it. Science measures the pH of the soil to achieve the same end. But this operation must not be regarded as necessary to confirm the farmers' conclusions; both realms must be accepted for what they are and a synthesis sought between the two.

From this synthesis emerges the guiding principles of agroecology, which does not seek to formulate solutions that will be valid for everyone but encourages people to choose the technologies best suited to the requirements of each particular situation, without imposing them. One of these principles, for example, is diversity; but diversity may assume various forms, such as an agroforestry system, polyculture, or crop rotation. What matters, I repeat, is not the technique but the principle: in this case the principle is that the selected kind of diversity will generate ecological processes in the system which will enable it to self-regulate and carry out autonomously operations such as nutrient recycling or pest and disease control.[27]

Agriculture and ecology are part of gastronomy because they help us understand where our food comes from and produce it in the best possible way—by simultaneously observing the principles of taste, respect for the environment, and biodiversity. The two disciplines are an extremely efficient compendium of forms of knowledge, both traditional and modern, which must be interrelated if we are to achieve maximum production in the most sustainable way possible. A gastronomy which is well-informed about agriculture and ecology and intercommunicates with them is a science that knows its own limitations, and will be able to find the natural resources to guarantee development in the most threatened areas of the planet without harming the environment. At the same time, it will be able to find a means of correcting the current implosion of the agroindustrial system.

2.4 On anthropology and sociology, or On identity and exchange

Food, being a primary cultural element, lends itself very well to the study of cultures and identities.

Anthropology is the science of culture, and as such it finds food a very fertile field of research, as the best representation of societies and the best means of interpreting their characteristics. There are some famous examples of such studies, from Claude Lévi-Strauss's *The Raw and the Cooked* to Marvin Harris's *Good to Eat: Riddles of Food and Culture*. In the same way, the study of gastronomy without an anthropological perspective omits the profound significance that food has for man and makes the mistake of not considering diet as an evolving *continuum*, but as a set of fixed rules that summarily identify the various cultures.

Sociology, for its part, studies the social life of people, groups, and societies (and therefore the identities of, and exchanges between, different societies and cultures, or how identities are formed and, in a gastronomic perspective, what dietary manifestation they have). As such, it provides an extensive body of data and analytical tools that are useful to gastronomy, and it can use gastronomy as a basis for its own research.

Anthropology and sociology help us understand the complexity of the choices that people make, and at the same time, in a historical perspective, they help us understand our present situation through the exchanges, references, and social conflicts that have defined gastronomic identities and food systems; they also help us seek possible ways of redressing the balance of the global system by anticipating its future trends.

They enable us to find out about the methods that man has used to survive, adapt to, and harmonize with his environment, and thus, in light of what is happening in the world today, reevaluate traditional knowledge and skills. In such a way, Lévi-Strauss, running counter to the methods of his predecessors, documented the vast amount of empirical knowledge that characterized nonliterate thought, in order to show that this thought was not just a matter of chance, so to speak, nor lacking in rationality. In order to achieve this, he may be said to have made considerable use of gastronomy.

The cosmology of nonliterate cultures shows, moreover, that ancient populations, though they lacked a scientific basis for their knowledge, understood the laws of the universe through constant empirical observation. For example, as far back as two thousand years ago, the Sami (see Diary 14) believed that the Earth went round the sun, long before Copernicus and Galileo developed their own theories about heliocentrism. Simple expedients devised to avoid starvation, or at least to make food shortages as pleasant as possible, also form part of this picture. Anthropology, together with ethnology, is concerned with the study of traditional knowledge, and often, because of its need to document that knowledge, is the only source we have on skills that have been lost.

Anthropology and sociology can also tell us why some foods are preferred to others, and they remind us of some fundamental laws which humanity seems to have forgotten:

> Even for an omnivore it makes sense not to eat everything that one can digest. Some foods are hardly worth the effort needed to produce and prepare them, some have cheaper and more nutritional substitutes, and some can only be eaten at the expense of giving up more advantageous items. Nutritional costs and benefits form a fundamental part of the balance—preferred foods generally pack more energy, proteins, vitamins, or minerals per serving than avoided foods. But there are other costs and benefits that may override the nutritive value of foods and make them good or bad to eat. Some foods are highly nutritious, but people spurn them because too much time and effort are needed to produce them, or because of the adverse effects they have on soils, animal and plant life, and other aspects of the environment.[28]

The simple expediency of not "having negative effects" on the environment should alert us to the fact that we are doing something wrong on this planet, that the costs are beginning to outweigh the benefits.

Anthropology and sociology are part of gastronomy because they are interdependent and interfunctional sciences, because they study human culture and can use gastronomy to prove their theories. Meanwhile, gastronomy, for its part, turns to these two disciplines to improve its understanding of food systems, of the history of nutrition, and of the knowledge of food production and processing that has been handed down within specific cultures.

2.5 On geopolitics, political economics, and trade, or On globalization

It has never been so clear as it is today that geopolitics, political economics, and trade must be an integral part of gastronomy. In what has been called the age of globalization, exchanges are multiplying in every direction, complexity is increasing, and our diet is strongly influenced by this. Moreover, trade seems to have become the new god: the expediency of consuming one type of food rather than another, which used to be linked to geoclimatic and economic factors, has gradually been replaced by the rules of the market. The models of traditional cooking, which once had to contend or harmonize with the physical limitations of territories and with the relationships that formed between different societies, are now on the verge of disappearing because of the emergence of a model where what prevails, after intense industrialization and the globalization of trade, is consumerism and detachment from the agricultural world.

The history of man can be reconstructed through a geohistory of taste, where general models of cuisine become dominant and come to characterize the various areas of the planet. These models are the result of the use of local resources, of the blending and collision of cultures, of the dominance of some over others following wars and various forms of colonization. Almost all wars have been waged because of a more or less openly avowed desire to appropriate fertile land as a potential source of nourishment or wealth. Some, for example, argue that even the conflict between Israel and Palestine is due not so much to religious factors as to a struggle, dating back to 1967, over the control of water sources in this extremely arid part of the world.

Nowadays, many of these wars are fought on the commercial level, with the agribusiness and food multinationals in the role that used to belong to the nation-states. It is no coincidence that the antiglobalization movement has developed strongly in connection with themes relating to agriculture and nutrition, first coming to public attention through the protests in Seattle during the WTO meeting of 1999. Half of the total world population is involved in agriculture, and the laws of global trade are putting terrible pressure on the economies of the poorer countries, which still have a significant agricultural component. The interference in those cultures by the seed multinationals grows ever stronger and more devastating, and it is supported by very aggressive commercial strategies and by a system of tolls and subsidies for production that create a serious imbalance in the world. The rich West produces too much, sold at excessively high prices; to defend itself against the competition of the poorer countries, the West creates insurmountable commercial barriers that impose artificial prices. The Western policy of subsidies for the quantity produced has brought the poorer economies to their knees and in effect financed the destruction of the planet. These subsidies (still very influential in the United States, though in Europe a recent review of agricultural policy is beginning to make the distortions of this system less pronounced) enable the farmers of the rich West, who practice an industrial kind of agriculture, to beat off the competition of the poorer countries, which can produce at a lower cost.

For many years, the effect has been to finance poor-quality production whose main aim was to keep costs as low as possible, regardless of how good the product was. The industrial agricultural model has been vigorously defended despite the fact that it has long been known to be unsustainable; the poorer countries have been pushed into an unrealistic pursuit of the same model of development, causing immense damage to biodiversity and the traditional cultures. These countries become the victims of dumping—that is to say, of invasion by the rich countries' surplus produce, which is subsidized at home and sold off at token prices, indeed often given away in the form of humanitarian aid. This process undermines local agricultural production, and it is because of such policies that in many areas of Africa, where the population is starving, the possibility of beginning to produce food or promoting local agriculture has gradually disappeared from the options of "development." What is promoted is a mendacious dependence on the rich world, which gives vast quantities of aid. The fact that the United States sends GMOs that have remained unsold because of the moratorium imposed by Europe on these products, or wheat, corn, and other grains with split seeds which are useless for sowing, says a lot about the donors' philanthropic intentions. And the fact that some African countries have begun to refuse this kind of aid confirms its relative uselessness and the detrimental effect that it has on local agricultural development.

Commercial priorities have come to dominate everything else, and the multitude of global injustices is almost infinite. A gastronome who has an ecological sensibility and who tries to promote forms of social justice through his choices cannot remain indifferent to a system of this kind, which is simply a global economic-financial pendant of the agribusiness model. As I have mentioned, this system has caused immense damage in the past and continues to do so: we must reject it out of hand.

In addition to providing the tools for an interesting historical account of how taste and food cultures are formed, geopolitics and economics thus make it possible to interpret the complex dynamics that underlie the present world system and to bring out all its injustices, contradictions, and paradoxes. Trade, for example, which according to Brillat-Savarin is the "search for the means of buying at the best possible price that which it [gastronomy] consumes and of selling at the highest possible profit that which it puts on sale," and which historically has been a prime cause of the meeting of cultures, has today become a tool of domination, or rather a weapon of conflict, in the context of a globalized world. The study of these dynamics, with regard to the world of food, is gastronomy, and the understanding of these dynamics provides a basis for defining the social sustainability of productive and commercial models, and the conditions in which such sustainability can be achieved.

2.6 On technology, industry, and know-how, or On methods of production

Traditional cultures have invented the most disparate methods of food processing and preservation, making the best possible use of the resources available to them. It is obvious, therefore, that the method of food production is a gastronomic subject, but the fact is worth repeating nonetheless, in view of what has happened over the last fifty years: a revolutionary process that has given rise to a dualism between traditional cooking and industrial methods of production.

Culinary techniques have gradually disappeared from homes, from the stock of widely shared knowledge. In many cases professional cooks are the only people who still possess this knowledge, this know-how that was formed over centuries of practice. Through industrialization, this ancient knowledge has been transferred to increasingly centralized places of production, and the production of our food has been delegated to those who are able to do it on a mass scale, using new and highly sophisticated techniques. (These techniques efface the traditional ones and cannot be replicated at home; a good example is the artificial flavoring industry.) This transfer of knowledge has deprived us of the know-how and skills we need to process our own food. There has been a growing predominance of industrial food technology over more traditional methods. Such methods, often dismissed because they were part of everyone's normal stock of cultural knowledge and were deemed unworthy of scientific attention, have faded almost completely away because others produce our food for us. For many today, cooking has become chiefly a matter of heating up something precooked and frozen.

The predominance of technology can be understood if we consider the current academic status of gastronomy compared to that which is accorded to the food technologies. It is the latter that are studied at the universities; students choose them so as to acquire specialist knowledge that will enable them to become valued employees of the food industry. In the university world, gastronomy has never been represented except in its more folk-loristic forms, or at most as the subject of anthropological and ethnographical research, whereas the food technology used by industry boasts high-powered specialists who teach at universities all over the world.

In reality, the fund of traditional knowledge on the subject of food processing—the set of simple acts of everyday preparation—is an extremely rich and valuable heritage. These acts are evident in every society that is prevalently agricultural, and they were equally important in the city, too, before the standardized models of the food industry became completely dominant. The tools and manual skills necessary to perform these acts are disappearing after centuries of practice, yet in many cases they prove irreplaceable. The great chefs themselves acknowledge this by risking the charge of overfussiness from those who are superficial about such matters, or by declaring their inability to perform certain apparently simple tasks in the kitchen.

A great master of the culinary art, Fulvio Pierangelini, who runs the Gambero Rosso restaurant in San Vincenzo, Versilia, confessed to me that he pays the closest attention to the manual skills of those who work with his raw materials. For it is the direct relationship established between the person who performs a simple operation and the material itself that shows the person's respect for that material and his ability to elicit the best organoleptic characteristics from it. Pierangelini told me, for example, of the time when he had once fired a young assistant after a few days' trial, even though he had previously worked in some excellent kitchens. When cutting fish, the boy simply would not move his hands in the way that Pierangelini had taught him. Either for convenience or out of sheer incompetence, he persisted in holding the knife at a completely different angle with respect to the working surface from the one he had been shown. Pierangelini was incensed, and after several reprimands eventually sacked him. What particularly infuriated him, he said, was that the young man defended his poor workmanship by saying that cutting was cutting, what difference did it make?

It would be interesting to ask for an opinion on which of the two men was right from a sushi chef, who does not dare to cut fish in the presence of customers until he has had years of training in the kitchen. Or we could just try to make sushi at home ourselves and observe the effect of our unskilled cutting on the flavor of the final product.

Often, moreover, this kind of knowledge was the exclusive property of women, as the principal occupants of the kitchen. Pierangelini tells me that in his kitchen no man, not even he, is allowed to clean and wash the salad and vegetables: this task is reserved for women, because he says they move in a different way from men. We may call it grace or skill, but the fact is that Pierangelini treats his older female assistants with utter devotion, and he told me this anecdote in a slightly despairing tone because one of them was soon to retire. He feared that nobody else would be able to prepare the vegetables for his kitchen as she did, her actions "mechanical and decisive, but with a grace and precision only possible for a person of great sensitivity."

The heritage of these movements, these manual skills, this unwritten and unwritable know-how, must be preserved, and some of the resources available for research should be dedicated to them, so that we can at the very least record them before they completely disappear. It is necessary, indeed urgent, to use all the available technologies (photography and computing, for example) to catalogue and store these manual acts and traditions in a kind of "skills bank."

It may be obvious that production techniques are an integral part of gastronomic science, but it bears repeating that modern gastronomy *must* concern itself with the oldest forms of knowledge, those practical and manual skills which I provocatively include here, under the heading "know-how," among the scientific disciplines: first of all with the aim of conservation, and secondly in order to revive or reproduce valid alternatives to the present unsustainable model, practicing at the culinary-productive level, too, that "matrix of dialogue between different realms" (official science and traditional knowledge) that Professor Altieri demands for agroecological theory. In effect, it is a question of studying all the methods of production and according them all equal dignity, so that we can abandon those that are most harmful to the human race and preserve the good ones that still have much to teach us.

2.7 On cooking and kitchens, or On the home and the restaurant

By cooking we mean the art of preserving, preparing, and cooking food. Some describe it as a form of language:[29] it has words (the products and ingredients), which are organized according to rules like grammar (the recipes), syntax (the menus), and rhetoric (table manners and behavior). Like language, cooking contains and expresses the culture of the person who does it; it is a repository of the traditions and identity of a group. It self-represents and communicates even more strongly than language, because food is directly assimilable by our organism: eating someone else's food is easier and more immediate than speaking their language. So cooking is the area *par excellence* of cultural interchange and combination.

The history of cooking was written in the recipe books of the aristocracy, a fact that has generated a false separation between gastronomy, perceived as elitist, and mere eating, aligned with the lower classes. In reality, the two things belong to the same sphere, since the cooking of the nobility has always drawn liberally on the popular, peasant, and lower-class tradition. At any rate, the aristocracy codified cooking through their chefs and through the works of history that have come down to us. Then, after 1789, with the French Revolution, the cooks left the palaces, and restaurants were born. Chefs became the repositories of "official" cooking. Alongside this official strand of the tradition, for at least two centuries people continued to practice in their homes an everyday kind of cooking that was open to the field and the kitchen garden, to the local market, to the small neighborhood shop. But now, even within the home, the most dramatic changes have taken place: industrialization has had a profound impact, globalization has brought a greater exchange of products and culinary models, and restaurant catering has become affordable to ever larger sectors of the population. Is it any surprise that we have bartered the everyday art of gastronomy for its monetized version? In the rich countries, kitchens in the home are less used than previously; people do not cook anymore, they buy food ready-made, whether in the form of prepackaged meals, lunch at a fast-food joint, or a sumptuous dinner in a restaurant that specializes in *nouvelle cuisine* or fusion cooking. It is not a matter of class—the evolution of social customs has distanced everyone in the industrialized West from their kitchens, whatever their background.

Even gastronomes—I myself am a good example here—have gradually abandoned the kitchen. In order to write his classic cookbook *La scienza in cucina e l'arte di mangiare bene* (Science in the Kitchen and the Art of Eating Well), the chef Pellegrino Artusi spent years in the kitchen aided by the faithful assistant Marietta, trying out all the recipes he collected; but the gastronome, since the days of Brillat-Savarin and Grimod de La Reynière, has come more and more to resemble a critic, indeed a judge. He enters a restaurant, does not even visit the kitchen, samples the final dish (the result of a long and complex procedure), and pronounces his verdict. I myself—I freely admit my deficiencies—am not a good cook. But I am aware of the respect and the scientific interest that culinary skill merits, and I know that I must take this into account if I wish to judge a dish in a restaurant; so I always make a point of asking to meet the chef and his team, of visiting the kitchen and watching the staff at work. Indeed, in light of the current situation around the world, even the cooks themselves deserve our efforts at preservation: whether they work at home or are employed in small traditional restaurants all over the world, such cooks possess recipes and culinary skills that must not be lost.

If we considered only the general situation, we might well conclude that cooking has died out; but in reality, it is only a question of retrieving knowledge and know-how that still exists, of learning it, supporting it, and replicating it. For globalization in cooking is in fact a big paradox.[30] In the past, the aristocracy pursued a certain kind of universalism; they could afford whatever they liked, they had access even to foodstuffs that were produced a long way away. Their cuisine was, or at least aspired to be, globalized, in the sense that, even though there might be countless local variants of a dish, the name and the main ingredients were always the same, shared at a national level. Globalization was a luxury of the wealthy.

Today, however, globalization, with its standardized industrial products, is within the reach of the middle and lower classes; but this advance has led to a drastic deterioration in our diet, and we eat food that has been mass-produced with little attention to gastronomic values. If you want to have a better diet nowadays, however rich or poor you are, you are forced to seek out local food and immerse yourself in nonglobal traditions. While modern globalization has favored the standardization of all the main culinary traditions, it has also generated new diversities and given new importance to the rediscovery of culinary identities. Local cooking, for example, is a fairly recent invention in the history of cooking, and it grows more attractive and important the more standardized the world becomes from the cultural point of view.

For many people, cooking—and the kitchen as the place where the activity takes place—is becoming an antidote to the lifestyles imposed by the dominant social models, a form of gastronomic resistance and protection of diversity.

Cooking, despite those who proclaim its death, is the main source of nutrition, identity, and perpetuation for a culture made up of thousands of individual people who repeat the same gestures and communicate with each other. However far the distance between those people, cooking is a matter of repeating actions, combining ingredients, inventing variants—it is the space of shared memory and identity.

Cooking is the mental place—as the kitchen is the physical space—of gastronomy. It is an area that is constantly evolving, and the only thing that threatens it is abandonment, which is a brutalization of our civilization that we simply cannot afford. We must give cooking back its rightful dignity and make it a subject of scientific research; gastronomes, and everyone else, must return to it, starting in their own homes. They must learn, if not the practical techniques of cooking, at least its theoretical importance, the incalculable value of the stock of cultural knowledge connected with it, and the awareness that without cooking, gastronomy is hardly possible. When I asked the chef Alain Ducasse what his definition of gastronomy was, he told me:

> Gastronomy is looking at a product and trying to respect its original flavor, the flavor of the people who cultivated, raised, or invented it, using the right method of preparation, the right duration of cooking, and the right accompaniment. The message of gastronomy must be clear to everyone and remain permeable so that we can appreciate what nature has given us. It is the respect for the product.

Gastromony can be attained only with good raw materials, of course, and with an approach to cooking that respects them. The message we receive from nature must remain "permeable" until the end: only cooking can achieve this.

2.8 *On the physiology of taste, or On sensoriality*

Taste—today a very overvalued word which adorns the titles of books, events, TV shows, and village fêtes because of its cachet—is primarily a matter of physiology. Although "taste" can indicate not only something that is good to eat but also something that is good to think (indeed, it is often used in this more "cultural" sense, as the outcome of the preferences of a social group), it is first and foremost one of our five senses. Together with the other senses, it enables us to taste and evaluate a food product in an almost objective, or at least comparative, manner. Certainly, a number of factors influence our perception of what tastes good or bad; taste is the knowledge of flavors extended to the entire heritage of an artistic and intellectual culture. But if we restrict the field to sensoriality alone, removing all the other admittedly interesting meanings of the word, there is no longer any power of discretion, and taste can be defined scientifically. This definition is based on the practice of tasting; an example is what happens with wine, where descriptive categories have been created for what we perceive with the senses of sight, smell, and taste. The same thing can be done with every kind of food, and this constitutes a firm scientific basis, which today can be said to have been completely defined and scientifically proved.

The most obvious and least "scientific" proof is an experience common to us all, deriving from the power (a power which has been scientifically demonstrated) of the gustatory-olfactory memory, the most persistent kind of memory in all human beings: there are flavors and smells that take us straight back to periods of our life that we had forgotten. I, for example, can well remember the aroma (not a particularly delicate one, but central to my Piedmontese gastronomic identity) that wafts through the air when slices of bread spread with *brus* are placed on the stove. *Brus* is a cream made by softening cheese and periodically stirring into it a little milk or rum. It is rarer than it used to be, as are the stoves and the practice of warming it on a slice of bread, but when I was a child I often had it for a snack, and the pungent smell is still etched on my memory more powerfully than any recent memory. The same is true of my predilection for the acid and the sour. In the warm months, my mother used to cook *giardiniera* (vegetable soup) and *carpione* (fried and marinated fish), both of which were based on vinegar, and now the taste is ingrained in my memory, unconsciously linked as it is to special, important experiences of my life—experiences I could not even describe without reference to my gustatory-olfactory memory.

Taste, as a sense, is the gastronome's principal tool, and it depends entirely on him. By this I mean that sensoriality is a capacity that needs to be trained, educated. The human sensorial universe in the present age has been impoverished as never before: artificial flavorings confuse and atrophy our senses, continuously raising the threshold of our perception and bombarding us with tastes and smells that do not exist in nature. Our senses, incomparable tools for a deeper understanding of the environment and of ourselves, have undergone a regression owing to the rhythms of life to which we are forced to conform, and which deprive us of many exquisite ways of tasting the world. Meanwhile, the stimuli multiply, and our perception becomes too selective, to the point where it will only accept the sensations which are necessary at that particular moment. But the senses can be re-educated, as I have mentioned, and this is the gastronome's mission.

I will go further: in a world where "sensorial deprivation leads to the dulling of our abilities to see, touch, taste, and smell," the training of the senses becomes "an act of resistance against the destruction of flavors and against the annihilation of knowledge."[31] It becomes a political act, for, once we are able to control and manage the mechanisms that regulate the transmission of stimuli and conditioning factors, we are also able to control and manage reality: the more vigilant our attention, the lower the risk of perceptual deception; and the richer our analysis of our perceptions, the greater our satisfaction and pleasure. The senses can become tools of choice, defense, and pleasure; they give new "sense" to our actions in all fields. The gastronome, from this point of view, may be seen as a privileged person who can discern and who, by his choices, which are guided by a sensibility immune to the distractions of industrialized society, can direct our future.

Recaptured sensoriality is the main, almost primitive, tool for orienting political action against a system in which the machine has become the real master: "Machinism produces counterfeit coin and tries to convince us that it is money. Laboratory knowledge does not reproduce life [and its flavors,] but its representation in world trade. Agroindustrial products are nothing but a machinic simulacrum of life, the result of the destruction of social relations in agriculture and the synthetic surrogate of exchange between man and nature."[32]

It is essential, therefore, that people receive a lifelong education in these matters, beginning in childhood and continuing throughout their lives. Such an education can only be provided and cultivated by the gastronome, for he alone, of all those who want to change the world, is aware that in order to achieve this goal it is possible to start from taste. One must learn to search for taste and to reject any simulacrum of it, such as artificial flavorings, which are the greatest—and also the more obscure— achievement of that system which is sapping our most natural human faculties day by day and which we must firmly reject.

2.9 On medicine, or On health and diet

Food in all societies, even the earliest ones, has always had a therapeutic function, a pharmacological component in the collective imagination. Cooking, as a mix of the benefits of nourishment and pharmacological compounds, has a long history, potentially associated with the evolution of the species. The balancing of nutrients in the past was achieved without the many calculations which the nutritional sciences are constantly publishing nowadays. In societies where the diet was poor in meat, for example, people got the protein they needed by eating insects (in Central America and in some parts of Africa, entomophagy is still quite widespread).

Often, however, learning from practical experience ("this food did me good when I was ill, so it can be used to cure or alleviate that particular illness with those particular symptoms"), traditional societies managed to construct an entire system made up of individual pieces of knowledge associating specific therapeutic properties to individual foods. Several examples come to mind: the indigenous Krahô people of the Brazilian *cerrado* had to fight hard[33] to recover the seeds of a particular variety of corn, *pohumpéy*, which has close links with their cosmology, but which also has a pharmacological function. This corn is said to be the gift that a goddess, the Star Woman, had given to their people: a legend tells how she appeared in a dream to a boy, showed him where he could find *pohumpéy*, and taught him how to grow it. That marked the birth of agriculture for the Krahô. But in addition to the symbolic value of this product, which had become extinct and was recovered from a germplasm bank in Brasilia, there is also the fact that, as the elders relate, the cobs of *pohumpéy*, when they are still small, green, and tender, were picked and used to make a soup believed to be energizing for pregnant women and their husbands. During the last few weeks of pregnancy and the first few weeks after the birth, the couple would feed exclusively on *pohumpéy* soup, which is also one of the foods reserved for frail children. Nowadays, this product is so rare that it is considered almost sacred, and its properties as a tonic are constantly praised.

In Europe, women were the repositories of pharmacological knowledge connected with herbs, until the Inquisition began to stigmatize them as witches; a vast heritage of knowledge disappeared with them, and only today, thanks to developments in herbalism, can we attempt to recover it. One only has to think of the medical school of Salerno[34] to realize that a good diet has always been regarded as the basis of good health. Even Brillat-Savarin and the early gastronomes laid down a particular order for individual courses, partly to enhance the pleasure of the meal, but also so that the body could prepare to absorb it in the healthiest way possible.

It is interesting to note that agricultural societies lose this traditional knowledge of diet and health more quickly than do hunter-gatherer societies, a loss which goes hand in hand with sedentarization, the concentration of the population, and documented links between malnutrition and disease. Sedentarization also brings with it the development of the medical and nutritional sciences. All this has, of course, reached its zenith in our affluent modern societies, where the obsession with a healthy diet is an increasingly evident factor. On the other hand, eating disorders have multiplied in recent years: the main causes of this, too, seem to be sedentary lifestyles and the dominant influence of the food industry, which has significantly reduced the variety and quality of our diet. Obesity is becoming a national problem in the United States, and in Europe as well, where the number of children who are overweight from early childhood is far greater than ever before.

In this very problematic context, where malnutrition and obesity are rife, and where cooking might at first sight seem doomed, the nutritional sciences appear to be flourishing. They are popular with a public obsessed with the desire to lose weight, to conform with media-imposed standards of beauty, to have a "healthy and balanced diet." Although researchers have studied the diets recommended by various nutritionists—whatever their creed, scientific orientation, or ideology—no study, whether theoretical or practical, has found any of them to be effective. The various slimming (low-calorie) diets, when subjected to rigorous scientific analysis, have all proved to be worthless, especially in the long term.[35]

Yet the public demands diets: it may seem a paradox, but it is the truth. In the United States, the amount of money spent on dietitians and dietary products already rivals that spent on food.

Many developing countries as well are beginning to encounter the problem of obesity and all the associated eating disorders which we in the West know only too well. And yet nobody attempts to adopt a different lifestyle or diet. The science of nutrition is regarded as a panacea and enjoys great prestige (a prestige which gastronomic science conspicuously lacks), even though it often shows dangerous signs of collusion with the world of the agricultural and food business, signs which ought to arouse a little skepticism.

Nevertheless, nutrition must be considered as a branch of gastronomy, for without a gastronomic perspective it cannot find a solution to the dietary problems of the modern world. A detailed study of diet—not a purely scientific study, but one supported by humanistic disciplines, from history to anthropology, and combined with a reevaluation of traditional knowledge—has a gastronomic perspective. If nutrition is used only to correct the effects that the agroindustrial model has on our health, it will inevitably make more mistakes and create further problems, with the enormous media interest that foments and supports it.

Gastronomy is therefore medicine to the extent that, as a complex discipline, it teaches us the elements of a correct diet:

variety, quality, pleasure, and moderation. In this case, too, a blend of traditional knowledge and modern medical science cannot fail to be beneficial.

2.10 On epistemology, or On choice

Epistemology is that part of philosophy which critically examines scientific knowledge by analyzing its language and methodologies and the way it organizes concepts into theories, establishing criteria for their validity. During the foregoing survey of the various gastronomic disciplines—most of which are only partly scientific according to the official definition, but in my opinion deserve full scientific status—I have on more than one occasion underlined the importance of recovering, cataloguing, and studying the traditional forms of knowledge and comparing them with the corpus of "official" scientific knowledge.

Epistemology, therefore, becomes a gastronomic discipline—or rather, the gastronome must adopt an epistemological approach—when this reference to forms of knowledge that are distinct from official science becomes inevitable. The science of the farmers, of the producing communities, of the fishermen, of the cooks, has the same dignity as the more established academic disciplines, and is a field of human knowledge—some would put it under the heading "consumer culture"—which must not be neglected. Indeed, a better understanding of it will enable us on the one hand to establish its validity, and on the other to bring it into critical and, if possible, functional contact with the other, more modern schools of scientific knowledge. In short, I hope that the "dialogue between realms" that is called for by Professor Altieri of the University of California at Berkeley (see Diary 10) will materialize, so as to make agroecology effective and fruitful. This must happen in all the fields of gastronomy, from the natural sciences to zootechnics and cultivation; from the methods of processing raw materials to the manual and instrumental technologies; from the various forms of exchange and contact between societies to cooking and medicine.

In the first place, then, the epistemological approach serves to break down the old intellectual prejudice that to discuss gastronomy and diet is to engage in second-rate scientific activity, if not in mere divertissement—that same prejudice which made Brillat-Savarin refuse to sign the first edition of *Physiologie du goût,* and which influenced all his successors.

Secondly—to strain the argument a little, perhaps—if epistemology helps us understand the validity of traditional knowledge, it should be considered an essential step on the way toward gastronomic truth. That is, it enables us to interpret the reality of food in the world and, on the basis of this interpretation, to make an even greater cognitive effort, employing our trained sensoriality and gastronomic knowledge, to decide what styles of behavior to adopt and what choices to make every day with regard to the act of eating. The study of gastronomic knowledge (or gastronomic science) is a methodological process that does not follow the classical dictates of the acquisition of knowledge but takes an intellectual approach; this approach is open to the extreme complexity that characterizes any food production chain, and thereby provides us with the tools we need in order to be able to choose.

Our choice of food, from another point of view, is the most powerful communicative tool that we possess. Our decision about what to buy and consume, in a world where everything is geared to profit, is the first significant political act we are able to make in our lives.

It is the gastronome's responsibility to become learned: not a botanist, not a physicist, not a chemist, not a sociologist, not a farmer, not a cook, not a doctor. All he needs is to know enough of these disciplines to understand what he eats. He must have some of the knowledge of each of those specialists, as far as food is concerned. And he must not be intimidated if experts look down on him as an amateur. Better to have a smattering of botany so that you can recognize a particular variety of plant, so that you know how, where, and by whom it was grown, how it was preserved and cooked, whether it can be bad for your health or not, and so that you can enjoy it more consciously. The alternative is the perfect biotechnologist, happy to eat a genetically modified organism that is harmful to farmers and the environment—a substance manipulated by the food industry, warmed up in a saucepan, and sadly lacking in taste.

The gastronome must be able to choose; that is his main "mission." He must be able to make correct choices, and he must understand all the complexities of the food production system. In the next chapter, therefore, I shall attempt a definition of quality—the quality that we must buy, study, promote, create, and teach. My aim in doing so is not to establish infallible rules, but to stimulate the reader to think about the power we have by virtue of the fact that we eat; and I hope to do this without denying or depreciating our natural propensity for pleasure and play. Indeed, I will start precisely from this element, taste: the good, which is the first and most immediate sensation that a food can give us. Striving for the good is the principal means we possess of promoting a kind of food production that is clean and fair—that is to say, sustainable.

CHAPTER III

QUALITY AS
AN OBJECTIVE

The word "quality," like "taste," "local," and "traditional," is one of the most abused terms in culinary literature. With the growing awareness among the public of the need for a healthy diet, "quality" is demanded and invoked for various reasons by everyone involved in agricultural and food production, and is widely used as a means of promoting a product.

The rise in popularity of the term is a fairly recent phenomenon, which came about mainly as a result of food scandals such as mad cow disease, dioxin-contaminated chicken, and various other dangers that have occurred periodically in the agricultural and food system since the late 1980s. Certainly, a more recent part of the credit—or blame?—for the spread of the word is undoubtedly due to the relative success of traditional products, generally produced with a heightened concern for the final result in terms of taste and originality. But it was the scandals in particular that opened the eyes of the average consumer (the recent success of certain "minor" producers, achieved in the face of current trends, proves this), shocking the general public because they entered homes, affected local farmers, and introduced fear and uncertainty—due to a profound lack of information—into the act of shopping. No media campaign in favor of quality would have been so effective, but soon the term became a feather to put in any cap, a term with infinite connotations that could be used in the most disparate contexts.

In the early 1980s, "quality" usually implied a concern with superior production methods and organoleptic characteristics, and was intimately linked with the idea of status, in accordance with a still very elitist concept of gastronomical knowledge. Toward the end of the century, however, the need to "democratize" the term after the food scandals (and the market success of the "local" and the "traditional") soon led to it acquiring a sense—warmly approved by the world of production—which in effect associates quality with hygienic-sanitary safety or at least equates quality with "local" and "traditional": "this product is not harmful to health, and does not kill, therefore it is a quality product"; or "this product is traditional in our nation and in this particular town, therefore it is a quality product."

This highly reductive concept is readily traceable to the intellectual tendencies imposed by technocratic and reductionist thought: when defining quality became a matter of urgency, people tried to regulate it on the basis of calculations or minimum quantifiable measures and requirements, which were often superficial. The most blatant example is provided by the European Union (EU), whose response to the demands prompted by the food scandals was to introduce an extremely restrictive type of regulation that had been under consideration since the early 1990s: HACCP (Hazard Analysis and Critical Control Points).

HACCP is a method first developed in the United States by NASA in 1959 to guarantee the quality of the food that was eaten in space programs; it was adopted by the EU as a way of controlling food production in 1994 and incorporated into Italian legislation in 1999. It consists of a set of norms and procedures for analyzing the risks of the contamination of products, from raw materials to the final product. It is a very restrictive and detailed method which, though possibly sustainable by the food industry with huge but proportionate investments, is impossible to sustain for small producers, especially those that use traditional or non-mechanized methods and tools of production. The main effect of HACCP has been an intolerable increase in red tape, a considerable rise in costs to meet standards, a standardization of production to the advantage of the food industry, and greater power of harassment for the controlling bodies. The vigorous opposition of some associations—Slow Food prominent among them—and of many small producers later induced the EU to soften its stance, allowing proportionate exemptions for those kinds of production that for structural reasons are unable to comply with these hygienic-sanitary criteria, which in fact only correspond to the characteristics of industrial methods of food production.[36]

This predilection for a quantitative idea of food quality—which had the immediate effect of equating quality with safety—went even further, producing more complex attempts to calculate and define quality. But these attempts were abandoned as soon as they came up against the infinite number of variables which the definition encounters. What characteristics must a cheese have in order to be considered a quality product? Must it be pristine, well-preserved, healthy, clean, fragrant, containing the right amounts of fat, salt, and dry residue? To the taste, it still might seem dull, even unpleasant: quality cannot be calculated; there is no such thing as objective quality.

But there is such a thing as comparative quality: must we therefore resign ourselves to relativism?

Certainly not. We can describe quality, and we can try to define it by looking for general requirements, criteria that are open to interpretation case by case. Quality is a complex concept, arising from the complexity of gastronomy itself and therefore from numerous parameters; we must accept it and turn it to our own advantage. The subjectivity of quality must be a cause of orientation, not of confusion.

We may begin by saying that quality is a commitment that is made by the producer and the buyer, a constant endeavor, a political act (that may seem a provocative statement, but I will explain the reasons behind it later), and a cultural act; and that in order to escape from the impasse of its relativity, quality demands a lifelong education in food and taste, as well as respect for the earth, the environment, and the people who produce the food.

Perhaps this can provide us with our general criteria, or at least with ones from which we can start, applying them during the phase of gastronomic choice, when we purchase a food product: the phase of the search—without any rhetoric—for taste, which involves three ideas. The latter are also the three essential preconditions which must be met before we can say that a particular product is a quality product and from which we may start to discuss personal or collective preferences, and therefore relative quality.

The three notions are *good, clean,* and *fair*—three mutually interdependent and indispensable concepts.

In my long experience as a gastronome, I have given hundreds of interviews both as a critic and as the president of Slow Food. In all these interviews, there have been very few occasions when the interviewer did not ask: "What's your favorite dish?" or "What's your ideal meal?" It is repeated like a kind of mantra, and it shows how often culture and gastronomic journalism become banal and concentrate reductively on two elements alone: recipes and recommended restaurants. I confess that I find the question very irritating, especially if I am trying to describe the complexity of gastronomic science in the interview. Over the years, however, I have learned to relax and not worry too much about it, replying that my preferences depend on the place and situation I find myself in. But the fact remains that the question is an irritating commonplace which does justice neither to the gastronome's curiosity nor to the seriousness of the subject.

What is no joking matter, at the level of personal tastes, is the gastronome's formative experience, which is highly individual and rooted in the childhood of each one of us. This is what makes the adventure of food wonderful, because for each of us it has a different point of departure, which can be traced back to the community and family into which we were born. I, for example, come from southern Piedmont, and began to learn about food in the postwar years, between 1949 and 1958, the period which has been recognized by the Italian National Institute of Nutrition as the time when Italians had the healthiest diet—not because people were affluent (they were not), but simply because of the quality of the food.

Coming from a family on the borderline between the working class and the lower middle class, my roots lie in a culinary tradition that derived from what can still be described as a subsistence economy, and of which my paternal grandmother was a representative. My grandmother's patience in producing food and teaching you to love it was very common among the women of those days, who could make profitable use of the scanty materials that they had at their disposal, preparing unforgettable dishes in conditions of great economic hardship.

That is why certain tastes have remained etched on my memory—the first tastes, always linked to particular moments, which remained vivid reference points for everything that came later.

I remember the afternoon snacks consisting of *soma d'aj*, a slice of bread spread with a clove of garlic and a little salt and oil, and toasted on the stove: too rich for a child at four o'clock in the afternoon. Nowadays, no one would ever dream of preparing such a snack, but that was my first experience of garlic, a food it is always difficult to persuade children to eat. Then there was Sunday lunch, which consisted of meat-filled ravioli (*le raviole*, in Piedmontese), the meat being in fact the week's leftovers. My grandmother liked to add rice to it, and the lightness of the pasta gave the dish a unique consistency and a richness of flavor you would never have expected from leftovers—a real Sunday feast.

There was another dish, which was the quintessence of poverty and which I have never seen anywhere else since: rice boiled in milk, which was the food of the evening, when you tried to make a virtue of necessity. And finally there was *rolatine*, thin scraps of meat rolled around a filling of eggs, vegetables, cheese, and breadcrumbs, and served with a typical Piedmontese *salsa verde*.

It is strange to see how all these dishes, which are part of my makeup, are rarely made any more, except in some restaurants that recreate the gastronomic tradition with scholarly accuracy. Those tastes are in my head, but I have seldom come across them in later years.

I feel the same dismay when I no longer find good bread on our tables, but odorless and tasteless white rolls, lacking the flavor I remember in those loaves made with sour dough and live yeast. Besides, a copious consumption of bread at meals is part of the history of Italian cuisine, whose roots lie in an agricultural society. I have always been amused by the fact that when I go to France people tell me that the Italians' idea of an hors d'oeuvre is bread and water. But it is part of our flesh and blood; today, I really miss good bread, and it is always a pleasant surprise to be served excellent bread with a meal. Many restaurants in California, for example, offer delicious bread.

Food changes with time and so do traditions, which are not immutable; but a gastronome's gustatory-olfactory memory is like a bank, a filing cabinet that preserves knowledge and flavors which accompany him through life. That is why a constant training of his sensoriality can only help the gastronome and the culture of which he is part: the more conscious this memory is, the less gastronomic knowledge will be lost in the future.

1. GOOD

Trying to define the concept of quality by saying that a product, in order to be considered a quality product, must be *good* does not solve the problem of relativism. "Good" is what one likes, and what one likes should be related to the sensorial sphere, which is strongly influenced by personal, cultural, historical, socioeconomic, and contingent factors. It is difficult to find objectivity in all this. In fact, however, it is by renouncing objectivity, the desire to establish a rule that is valid for everyone, that one can arrive at an understanding of what is good. What is good in gastronomy is good if two conditions hold: first, that a product can be linked with a certain naturalness which respects the product's original characteristics as much as possible; secondly, that it produces recognizable (and pleasant) sensations which enable one to judge it at a particular moment, in a particular place, and within a particular culture. What is good for the present writer is not necessarily good for a twenty-year-old Londoner, a Mongolian shepherd, a Brazilian samba dancer, or a Thai doctor, let alone for a Masai from Tanzania. And in a hundred years, if I could still be here to taste it, it might not be good for me either.

In defining what is good, two kinds of subjective factors are crucial: *taste*—which is personal and linked to the sensorial sphere of each one of us—and *knowledge*—which is cultural and linked to the environment and to the history of communities, techniques, and places.

1.1 Sensoriality

The knowledge of the senses is scientific, in the classical sense of the term—that is to say, it has an objective basis, though a very weak one—because it is the way we perceive through sensoriality: it is a physical, physiological fact, which is natural in a healthy person.

The study of the human body on the one hand and the decoding of tasting techniques on the other have made it possible to explain how our senses function, how perceptual activity occurs and how it becomes cognitive. The tastes, the colors, the textures perceptible to the touch, the sounds, and the primary smells have all been identified and described.

The serious tasting of a food product, before one expresses a value judgment on it, passes through the most meticulous description of its characteristics: visual, olfactory, tactile, and gustatory. Some perfectionists even take pains to explain the influence of the sense of hearing on the total experience of taste. It has to be said that this approach can be described as a kind of *aesthetics* of eating and drinking, which already introduces a cultural element,[37] but the point of departure remains objective; only the value that is subsequently given to this or that taste, to this or that smell, changes.

The history of cooking comes to our aid to explain how the concept of the good is variable and how it has changed profoundly over the course of our history, completely overturning judgments. The ancient Romans were exceedingly fond of *garum*, a sauce made from fish entrails steeped in oil and various spices, a condiment we would abhor if it were still produced today; and yet, a very similar one is very common and much appreciated in present-day Thailand. There have been periods in history when the sour triumphed, others when the sweet was preferred, others still when the sweet, salty, and sour were used simultaneously; there have been periods when spices and artifice with respect to natural taste were synonyms of good, and others when a stronger need was felt for the final dish to respect as closely as possible the original taste of the raw materials.

At any rate, this variability, which we might describe as "evolutionary," and which is always linked to environmental conditions, does not mean that there is no objective way of recognizing *flavors*, the sensorial basis of all our approaches to food. And if we take the historical perspective, this basis has never been so much under threat as it is today. Human sensoriality is attacked by the multiplication of stimuli, by the diminution of the amount of time we have to select and perceive them, and by certain methods of industrial production which alter the natural flavors and end up deceiving us, indeed atrophying our overexposed and increasingly ill-educated senses.

Re-educating the senses and keeping them in constant training becomes the principal gastronomic act, the primary and indispensable task that enables us to recognize quality. If we cannot identify *flavor* on the basis of objective data, we cannot achieve *knowledge*. In this way we lose *pleasure*, our freedom of choice, and any chance of directly or indirectly influencing the decisions of producers. In so doing, we renounce quality from the outset and are compelled to trust those who sell it to us as such.

But it would be wrong to trust them too much; from this point of view, our regained and educated senses have a very important political role. The coarsening of our senses is a surrender to the ruling model, which does not want us to be pleasure-loving, satisfied people but unfeeling cogs in the juggernaut propelled toward profit (and the grave). The dulling of the senses to which we are subjected is both a consequence and a contributory cause of the proliferation of a system, a mode of thought and production, which has nothing in common with what food ought to be. Reappropriating the senses is the first step toward imagining a different system capable of respecting man as a worker of the land, as a producer, as a consumer of food and resources, and as a political and moral entity. To reappropriate one's senses is to reappropriate one's own life and to cooperate with others in creating a better world, where everyone has the right to *pleasure* and *knowledge*.

1.2 Taste

Taste is both flavor and knowledge, *sapore* and *sapere* in Italian: the alliteration of the two terms says a lot about the close connection that exists between the perceptual and cultural spheres. Taste changes according to whether you are rich or poor, whether there is abundance or famine, whether you live in a forest or in a metropolis. But for everyone, taste is the right to transform their own daily sustenance into pleasure.

This natural tendency has not always corresponded to criteria of cheapness with respect to costs and benefits: it may be a matter of expediency, as Marvin Harris maintains, but eating a particular kind of food does not necessarily mean that one appreciates it, as Jean-Louis Flandrin has pointed out.[38] The rich always seem to have taken *expensiveness* as the main criterion of their culinary choices:[39] to them, the rarer, and therefore the more costly, the product, the better it is. The greater diffusion of wealth nowadays—if not in the absolute sense, at least in the sense related to the cost of food—combined with the sensorial ignorance that is becoming ever more widespread, have also led to the criterion of expensiveness, only now it is inversely proportional to, and more unconscious than, elitist ostentation, but equally inexpedient: the cheaper a product is, the more I eat it, never mind if I deprive myself of pleasure and if it does damage to me, to the ecosystem, and to those who produce it.

But leaving aside all these anthropological and economic considerations, taste remains the crucial factor in establishing the goodness of a particular food. Its formation depends on the culture and the economic situation, and in light of these factors, it is the gastronome's task to succeed in defining what is good for the world of today.

As I have already said, however, it is not easy to arrive at a definition that is "good" for everyone: the variety of factors that are involved makes generalization difficult. The study of what is good, therefore, necessarily restricts the field to a single culture and a single social group. It sets limits (spatial, cultural, and social) and confronts us with all the complexity of multidisciplinary gastronomic science. But this very complexity and this cultural diversity, if accepted fully and open-mindedly, can enable us to clear away many factors which are unimportant (and very relative), so that we can single out those elements that occur in all cultures, a common point of departure. One of these elements might be, for example, a preference for the artificial or for the natural, which I consider to be a good starting point. Other rival factors belonging to other contexts will be superimposed on macrocriteria of this kind.

Another preliminary remark should be made: in order to develop these arguments, I will refer to the history of our taste here in the West, but I would like to state clearly at the outset that I totally reject Eurocentrism and any suggestion that our gastronomic culture is superior to others.

I start from "us" simply because we have more historical sources at our disposal, and many other scholars have given detailed descriptions of these dynamics. It has been demonstrated, for example, that Western history has been characterized by a cyclical swing between the artificial and the natural. Artifice was preferred in ancient Roman, medieval, and Renaissance cuisines, when cooking was perceived as a combinatorial art whose purpose was to change the natural taste of food as much as possible. But to delve less far back in time, the same alternating prevalence of the artificial and the natural is found even in the more recent development of *haute cuisine*; in the mid-1970s, there was a new vogue for *nouvelle cuisine*, which put the technical ability of the chef before all else as the key element in the success of a great dish, a dish that could be considered good. During this historical phase, the raw material was depreciated in its importance with respect to the good: according to the supporters of *nouvelle cuisine,* even the worst point of departure could be transformed into something exceptional by the technical ability and creativity of the cook.

After only a decade, in the mid-1980s, the popularity of new chefs such as Alain Ducasse inspired a new school whose aim was essentially the quest for excellent raw materials, which it held to be the only indisputable factor on which the chef's ability can legitimately intervene, to present the originality of the flavors in all their splendor. Then came the Spanish school led by Ferran Adrià, who with an injection of flamboyant and highly technical creativity reintroduced artifice to the kitchen: consistencies which change and cannot be traced back to the original appearance of the ingredients, flavors which do not correspond to appearances or smells. This continual and increasingly provocative game found intellectual justification in the work of Adrià, the only true innovator of the school (to call him a genius would not be an exaggeration), but became an exercise in sterility and bad taste in the hands of most of his followers.

Today, there is a continuing debate between this trend toward the technicalizing of cooking and the theories of those who favor a revival—or an adaptation to modern tastes—of traditional cooking. The traditionalists look to the work of those chefs who have in some way been inspired by these traditional cuisines in the sincerity with which they attempt to treat the original and natural tastes of the products. The tension between these two worlds is great, and the antagonism is exacerbated by the exigencies of a world so global in thrust that it is in danger of self-destruction.

It is increasingly obvious that any movement in a certain direction in a society like ours immediately prompts an opposing movement. When fast food became universal, Slow Food found its raison d'être; when globalization exercised its homogenizing power over taste, at once reactions sprang up which regarded localism and diversity as a value. If artifice comes into fashion, there is immediately a revival of the "natural" school. And in the midst of all this, the exchanges and amalgamations grow more and more uninhibited: fusion cuisine, for example, which blends together different products and culinary traditions purely on the basis of flavors, defying all territorial and cultural boundaries, can either lead to complete chaos (con-fusion), which completely distorts the value of the raw materials, or have the positive effect of introducing new cultural stimuli into the evolution of collective taste, spreading the knowledge of new products by means of respectful and pertinent combinations.

In this chaotic and rapidly changing situation, it is important to take up a position in favor of "natural" taste: for in the welter of stimuli that surrounds us, taste must first and foremost be clearly identifiable, both as *flavor* and as *knowledge*. Rejecting artifice for artifice's sake is an act of responsibility, a summons to go back to reality. Few artifices can justify a knowledge which is so great as to eclipse flavor (as in the case of Adrià).

1.3 Naturalness

Bearing in mind the characteristics assumed today by almost all agricultural food production of the industrial type—which is very influential on and influenced by technicalized and "unnatural" thought—and leaving aside any discussion of the validity of the techniques at the center of the debate, there remains today the question of raw materials and respect for them. This is the first factor in discussing the good.

Raw materials and respect for them: these are the minimum conditions on which to construct an axiom whereby the goodness of a product is proportional to its naturalness. The natural integrity of the raw material is what makes possible the cultivation and perception of the good.

At this point, we need to clarify what we mean by *natural*. Here we are discussing a general system, the method of production in its entirety. Natural means not using too many elements that are extraneous and artificial with respect to the system / environment / mankind / raw material / processing: no additives and chemical preservatives, no artificial or supposedly "natural" flavorings; no technologies that subvert the naturalness of the process of working, raising (in the case of livestock), growing, cooking, et cetera. The raw materials must be healthy, whole, as free as possible from chemical treatments and intensive procedures. They must be treated with processes that are very respectful of their original characteristics. The quality of a cheese, for example, is intimately linked with the quality of the milk that is used, and the milk will be good to the extent that the feed given to the animal that produced it was good. The same goes for meat, which will be good if the breeding of the animal has respected the criteria of naturalness: no growth accelerators, no hypercaloric or antibiotic-laced fodder. The animals should lead a stress-free life. Great respect should be paid for their well-being. In other words they should lead as "natural" as possible a life while they are being raised: adequate space if they are kept in stalls—but preferably they will be put out to pasture; very short journeys, made only when necessary and without them being crammed into trucks; no violence. It is not just a question of not being cruel to animals—all this is also a guarantee that the final product will be better: stress and trauma have a significant effect on the sensory qualities of meat.

But to what extent can human technology be reconciled with "naturalness"? Every agricultural technique, even the most archaic, introduces an element of artifice into nature. The same can be said of transformation (whether by cooking or other processing method), for it is true that with absolute naturalness the process of producing our food would not be "cultural": our diet would not be very different from that of animals, which eat what they find in nature without modifying it.

In this case, as in other areas of life, common sense should prevail: a technique is natural if it respects nature, does not abuse it, does not waste it, does not irreparably alter its balance. From this point of view, one may cite the example of wine production: is using a *barrique* to enhance its flavor in the cellar natural? It is certainly more natural than a concentrator, which alters the biochemical values of the grapes produced that year.

The *barrique* is a cellar technique that does not alter the wine's "naturalness." The same is true of thinning out in the vineyard (the technique of eliminating some bunches of grapes to concentrate the sugars in the remaining ones and thereby improve the quality of the grapes at the expense of quantity): this could be seen as an attempt to alter the productive season by external intervention. Yet thinning out is certainly more natural than the use of a concentrator or chemical treatments on the plants, for it is part of a process, a human know-how which is consistent with the "naturalness" of things, and it does not compromise production—indeed, it improves it without putting too much stress on the soil and the vegetation. A similar comparison could be made between, on the one hand, the techniques of cross-fertilization and varietal improvement through selection (the first is used in botany, the second by farmers and nurserymen after each harvest), and, on the other hand, the creation of hybrids invented for productive reasons or, even worse, the creation of genetically modified organisms—for the same productive purposes. (Surely the reader does not believe the lie that GMOs will solve the problem of world famine? But we will return to this point later).

This, then, is another essential prerequisite in our quest for the good: the product must meet the criteria of naturalness throughout the production process which brings food from the field to our tables.

1.4 Pleasure

The good is what we like. Pleasure has always been the gastronome's joy and torment. On the one hand, it is undeniable: if we strive for the good, we do so in order to experience, and enable others to experience, culinary pleasure. On the other hand, it is evident that those parts of Europe where a gastronomic culture has developed are the same ones that have most strongly felt the influence of the Catholic religion and whose dominant moral code rejects pleasure and associates it with vice, sin, and damnation. At the same time, the militant characteristic of certain political ideologies has considered the quest for gastronomic pleasure as succumbing to one of the worst bourgeois vices.

The enjoyment of food, which is constantly sought with the utmost ingenuity even where food is in short supply, is a physiological, instinctive matter, but one that is somehow rejected by our society. Gastronomy has not attained the status of a science, nor even really been taken seriously, because it is a subject that concerns pleasure.

This underlying problem has impeded the quest for the good, and has been a perfect accomplice of that industrial process of food production that has depreciated the importance of quality so much that it has almost disappeared (or merged with different concepts, such as hygienic-sanitary safety); as a result most people have become accustomed to highly artificial aromas, tastes, and sensations and are unable to choose the good because they cannot recognize it. The rejection or concealment of culinary pleasure has meant that the cutting of the umbilical cord that tied us to the soil and its fruits has been painless for most of us. Yet that break has separated producers from consumers, excluding the latter from any phase of the production process during which taste is created, flavor can be respected, and knowledge is fundamental.

The pleasure principle is fundamental. The pleasure principle is natural: everyone has a right to pleasure, as we saw earlier. To reaffirm this principle unambiguously and without any psychoanalytical implications is in the first place an act of civility. Since pleasure is a human right, it must be guaranteed for everyone, so we must teach people to recognize it, to create the conditions whereby "naturally" good products are producible everywhere.

This aim immediately eliminates the erroneous idea that gastronomy is the prerogative of a wealthy elite and that it must be in some way separated from food per se. That is like saying that only those who can afford it have a right to pleasure, and that everyone else, the poor, must simply eat to keep themselves alive and cannot experience pleasure.

This is not the case, and pleasure is always linked, indissolubly, with knowledge, which is itself another right: knowledge of the sensory characteristics of a product both when it is considered a raw material and after it has been processed; knowledge of the process that transforms it, so that we can appreciate its validity; knowledge of the characteristics of products that are similar but of different provenance and made with different techniques; knowledge of ourselves and our sensibilities, which must be communicated and shared with others.

Pleasure sought and expressed is contagious. It restores all the body's vitality and stimulates the intelligence to go beyond the rules of the old gastronomic code; it is a challenge to all those food-related disciplines (such as nutritional science) which often declare, in their inward-looking way, that they can do without it, whereas in fact without it they would have no raison d'être. Pleasure should be taught to children, adults, and the aged all over the world, because it is the only thing that gives meaning to the daily work of the new gastronome. It must never be introspection closed within the personal sphere, but rather a conscious philosophy of life which permeates and guides every gastronomic act, from cultivating to eating, from shopping to cooking, from the study of the food system to scientific research and development programs for those parts of the world where food is scarce.

Pleasure in this sense is a philosophy of the good, which works for the good and knows how to enjoy it.

1.5 The good as an aim
Because it is subjective, the good can be used as an instrument of division between social classes and peoples; and also of cultural division on the part of those who have an interest in the good not becoming too well known, or of those who, although their intentions are noble, believe that their "own" good is the "only" good and that it is applicable to everyone.

If I say that I seek the good, what I mean is that I seek what is good for me, what is good according to my culture, but at the same time I hope that everyone all over the world will find what is good for their cultures.

The Italians, for example, have many traditional dishes based on rabbit, but to many Americans eating rabbit is an inhumane and disgusting act, because the animal is regarded as a pet, like a dog. It is hard to explain to an American that the wild rabbit of Ischia, if bred in the traditional way, acquires superior sensory characteristics. For many Americans, rabbit is not even edible! The same can be said of the *brus* which I mentioned earlier: not even the inhabitants of other parts of Piedmont would consider this product good, with that smell which many would describe as a stink! Perhaps it is not objectively good, but it is part of my culture, of my memory, and there are techniques for making it better or worse. Young people, for example, even those from southern Piedmont, where *brus* is still produced—though only in very small quantities—no longer have the right cultural background to appreciate it. They can, however, be trained to appreciate it by understanding the reasons why it is produced, why it acquires certain sensory characteristics, and which are the right ones; and all this because it belongs to the culture they were born into. But you cannot force them to eat it; it is a taste that is dying out, for tastes do evolve through history.

When I met some entomophagous women from Burkina Faso who dry certain larvae in the way they learned from their mothers, because in such a poor country insects and larvae are a readily available source of protein, they gave me a little bag of those caterpillars; out of politeness, but also out of curiosity, I tried one. Objectively speaking, I did not find anything that corresponded to my categories of "good" (though when I was served some similar larvae, fried, in Mexico City I found them delicious). To my personal taste, those insects are bad, but since they are important for that culture—they are part of the tradition, they meet the criteria of naturalness, their consumption helps agriculture because they are parasites, and what is more they improve the diet of the *burkinabé* (who love them)—I *must* say that they are good. Just as *brus* is good and the wild rabbit of Ischia, which is almost extinct, is good. This is the absolute relativity of the good: according to culture, according to "natural-ness," according to sensory characteristics.

Taking this relativity *in toto*, the concept may therefore mean in the first instance respect for other cultures, for diversity. This respect must guide every contact we have, every intervention we make in order to support or exchange with others, every tasting of food we make when we are in another country. No one has the right to judge someone else's food on the basis of their own "cultural" taste: if we accept the description of food as a language, it becomes a means of communication, and in order to judge it we must learn to recognize the categories of the good which have codified it, as a language, in that particular culture. We must learn other culinary languages.

This respect is difficult to put into practice and is the first obstacle and source of error when we try to organize international interventions to protect or support products, agricultures, or social groups connected with food. Usually, the nongovernmental organizations, the associations and institutions that work in these fields, are the products of Western culture and must not presume to impose their mode of thought—their taste—on others. They cannot even afford to do it in good faith. Even Slow Food, which through its international Presidia strives to defend small producers all over the world, finds it very difficult and makes a great effort to learn about the cultures where it intends to operate. If we strive to promote sustainability, naturalness, and local tradition, we also work to promote quality, and if we start from an erroneous concept of the good, we will fail.

In conclusion, the good as an objective has a political connotation. In order to reappropriate reality, we must take two important steps: recover our sensoriality as the founding act of a new way of thinking and acting or reacting; and gain respect for other cultures by learning to understand other people's categories (categories necessary for recognizing the good). These steps can help us to communicate, to work together to redeem food-producing communities, and, ultimately, to perceive reality through our senses as a *great network* of *flavors* and *knowledge*.

This global reality must be matched by an act performed at the most local level: eating in our own homes. This act of survival is aware of the good to the extent that it is aware of the planetary diversity that surrounds it. Although this act cannot have the benefit of omniscience, it starts from the sharing of criteria for making a "good" choice within a complex reality, which is accepted as such. The good is an aim, for quality is the aim of a new and universally shared sensibility or sensoriality.

1.6 Is it good?

The first of the three indispensable and interdependent prerequisites (good, clean, and fair) for a quality product is therefore that it be "good"—good to the palate and good according to the mind. The good has superior sensory characteristics, the best ones that can be obtained while respecting a criterion of naturalness. It will be the new gastronome's task to respect these characteristics, to learn to recognize them, to produce them or encourage others to produce them according to the culture in which he lives, and to prefer them always.

This is a political task. The purpose of politics is to improve the quality of life, and the good has the same function. If anyone should object that politics is a serious matter, that it has nothing to do with these questions, I would reply that the good, too, is a very serious matter. This is no heresy; there is nothing to be ashamed of.

Good is respect for others and for ourselves, striving to ensure that it becomes a right for everyone is part of our civilizing mission. Reaffirming the good must lead to respect for the earth and for its different cultures: we are talking about happiness. If anyone is alarmed to see how democratic the good can be, that is not the gastronome's problem. If this reaffirmation of pleasure offends the *bien pensants* (who, however, take their own enjoyment selfishly and irresponsibly and never renounce pleasure), that is not our problem. Nor will it ever be, at least until the *good, flavor, knowledge*, and *pleasure* are denied us, withheld in the name of that fear and offense or, more dangerously, in pursuit of profit. Should that happen, then the gastronome will indeed be forced to intervene. We are talking about happiness: happiness for the earth and for its inhabitants.

{**DIARY 9**} THE INDIAN PRAWNS

On December 27, 2004, the world awoke to pictures of a disaster of apocalyptic proportions. A powerful earthquake a few kilometers off the coast of Sumatra had caused a huge tidal wave, which had struck thousands of kilometers of coast in Indonesia, Bangladesh, India, Sri Lanka, and even East Africa. Hundreds of thousands of people were killed, towns razed to the ground, and a wasteland of ruins was left where previously there had been human settlements. Human lives were destroyed, societies torn apart, cultures threatened; the losses were incalculable. The rest of the world at once showed great solidarity; aid for the victims was mobilized on an unprecedented scale. Once the emergency was over, people began discussing the future of the areas affected—tourist resorts, coasts inhabited by simple fishermen and farmers, places where the local population, already beset by numerous problems, had to start all over again.

The debate about how to use the aid from the rich West was very intense in the months following the disaster, and for our part, to clarify our ideas on what needed to be done, Slow Food decided to hold a public debate, comparing two different points of view, two different visions of the world. The East and the West between Nature and Food was the title of the event, and it took place in Turin on February 14, 2004. We invited two friends to lead the discussion: Enzo Bianchi, prior of the monastery of Bose in northern Piedmont, and Vandana Shiva, the Indian scientist and activist.

The debate that evening sought answers, ranging over a variety of questions from our relationship with the supernatural forces that influence earthly actions to the culture clash in the tourist resorts that had been ravaged by the tsunami. The debate was of a very high level, and I was particularly struck by the opening words of Shiva, which were brutally direct and provocative:

> The effects of the wave that struck the coasts were mainly the fault of the human race. The coasts, bereft of their natural defenses because of the construction of tourist villages and the destruction of the mangrove forests for agroindustrial purposes, have been left completely exposed. As a result hundreds of thousands of lives have been put at risk. The principle of human responsibility toward nature has been disregarded and we have been hit with unprecedented force.

A responsible attitude to the environment characterized by a sacred respect for nature, for other human beings, and for future generations: this noble philosophy is part of everyday life in those countries, and is observed in agriculture and in human relationships of all kinds, but it has been suffocated by the irruption of a different culture and different methods of production.

Shiva told us a story of incredible "mal-production," which is in danger of being repeated with even more disastrous consequences now that reconstruction is underway. In many coastal areas affected by the tsunami in India and Bangladesh, intensive prawn farms have been created which have devastated the existing ecosystems, with serious consequences for the lives of the local inhabitants.

In the early 1990s, promising rapid development, huge profits, and the creation of new jobs, the experts of the World Bank managed to convince the Indian government that intensive prawn farming would put an end to centuries of poverty and of small-scale subsistence economy along six thousand kilometers of coastline. Prawn farming seemed to be the panacea which, under the far-sighted direction of the World Bank, would guarantee India lasting prosperity.

But these farms occupy vast areas. Within a few years, thousands of hectares of fertile soil, where the farmers had previously cultivated simple but diverse crops—especially rice—for their own needs, were transformed into huge open-air basins. Filling them requires a large amount of fresh water, so large that it has drained the water-bearing strata below the nearby villages. They also need a certain amount of seawater, which, in time, penetrates the soil, rendering it unfit for use in the short term.

The prawns are given massive doses of antibiotics to protect them from the diseases to which they are most susceptible, because they are living in extreme conditions: the population density in those basins is far too high. The antibiotics also serve as growth accelerators and, mainly for this reason, are overused. Moreover, the prawns are sprayed every day with the right quantity of chemicals to balance the artificial conditions of the ecosystem in which they live. This treatment of course requires a constant supply of water, which, for the sake of economy and simplicity, is then discharged into the sea.

In addition to the damage that has been done to agriculture, therefore, the fishing industry has also been crippled. The polluted water, which is rich in nitrates and nitrites from the prawns' excrement, accelerates the decline of the mangrove forests, which were already seriously depleted by the installation of the prawn farms. The presence of mangroves is extremely important in these areas because they protect the coast against the force of the sea (significantly, the tsunami did less damage along those parts of the coast that were still protected by the mangroves) and provide a refuge for the fish, which, once they are deprived of their natural habitat, either die or move elsewhere. The fishermen, who used to work inshore, are forced to buy deep-sea fishing boats—if they can afford them—and go further out to sea in order to catch anything.

The result? Widespread ecological damage, villages reduced to desperate straits, and widespread unemployment. A basin for a prawn farm employs two people, in an area which previously guaranteed work, year round, to 120 rice-growers. What is more, the prawns are intended for the markets of the United States, Europe, and Japan, which in recent years have been inundated with tons of these crustaceans. It should be mentioned that prawns were produced on the Indian coast even before the introduction of intensive farming, but in those days they were rotated with the growing of rice, a rotation that refertilized the soil ecologically (with unpolluted excrement) and also made use of the soil, which would otherwise have been left fallow for a year. Consumption was mainly local, but that is no longer the case: the local people, now jobless, cannot afford the expensive "industrial" prawns, a food which they once produced in harmony with nature for their own subsistence.

In the last few years, two disciples of Mahatma Gandhi, Krishnammal and Jagannathan, have been giving voice to the protests of the coastal population, which were being ruined by the aggressive invasion of these farms even before the tsunami. The World Bank, for its part, has already planned to rebuild the flooded farms—indeed, to enlarge them. I have no doubts about which side to take, and Shiva's story—published in Italy by Laura Coppo in her book *Terra, gamberi, contadini ed eroi* (Earth, Prawns, Farmers, and Heroes)—is another example of how a failure to respect local cultures and thousand of years of sustainable production can only worsen the lives of those we claim to be helping.

Moreover, failing to respect nature can be very risky: when nature rebels with such violence, whether or not it is a coincidence, technocratic man is always the first to aid in the destruction.

2. CLEAN

The second prerequisite for a quality product is that it should be *clean*. "Clean" is a far less relative concept than "good," though equally complex. Clean, too, corresponds to a criterion of naturalness, but in a different sense, or at least in a different conceptual development from that which we have described in the case of good. Naturalness here is related not to the intrinsic characteristics of the product, but rather to the methods of production and of transport: a product is clean if it respects the earth and the environment, if it does not pollute, if it does not waste or overuse natural resources during its journey from the field to the table. To use a more technical term, a product is clean to the extent that its production process meets certain criteria of naturalness, if it is *sustainable*.

It is around this word, "sustainable," that the definition of clean revolves. *Sustainability*, too, may be considered a very relative concept (but we must be able to calculate costs and benefits in order to establish exact rules: often the pollution resulting from production is accepted only because the real environmental costs are not known, or underestimated), so a *limit* must be set. The limit, in this case too, is primarily dictated by common sense, at least when it cannot be precisely calculated.

Finally, we should note the interdependence of the two concepts "clean" and "good" (and also of "fair," but we will come to that later): respect for the criterion of naturalness is the basis of both these principles, and there is a reciprocal relationship between them. A soil that is neither stressed nor polluted will yield products that have superior sensory characteristics; healthy air will make possible a better processing of the products. Giving the right balance to an ecosystem will help to reduce production costs and to fulfill the potential of any raw material.

2.1 Sustainable

What do we mean by "sustainable" in the context of food? Which is more sustainable—a crate of organic Brazilian mangos imported by ship, or the bread made by the local baker two blocks away from home? In order to be able to judge the sustainability of food products, we need to know the ecological consequences of the actions carried out during their journey from the land to the table. We must ask ourselves whether a particular food is healthy and safe, whether it has been produced in order to satisfy the needs of those who consume it (sustainable *good*), and whether its production and processing guarantee jobs and fair means of support (sustainable *fair*).

A product will be clean to the extent that it is sustainable from the ecological point of view. So in order to be able to assess all the effects that its production and processing have on the environment, we need a large and diversified body of knowledge. We need to know whether the varieties used are among the strongly commercial ones that reduce biodiversity; whether the techniques of cultivation and farming impoverish the soil with pesticides or excrement from animals "pumped up" with fodder and drugs; whether the processing has been carried out in factories or in artisanal workshops that do not pollute and do not use polluting products; whether the means of transport the product has been subjected to were too long or involved producing a high level of atmospheric pollution; and whether we ourselves harm the environment in obtaining or buying them. It is not easy; the judgment of sustainability requires a process of investigation and reflection that we as consumers have never before been required to go through.

To return to the example of the mangos and the bread: at first sight, the Brazilian mangos might seem to be less sustainable than the bread, simply because they come from a long way away. But they may not be: they are certified as organic products, so presumably no pesticides have been used in producing them; they have been transported by ship (and from the port to our homes perhaps by train), which pollutes much less than a plane or a truck. The bread, on the other hand, may have been made with flour from intensively cultivated wheat, which may have been transported for many kilometers on a truck before reaching the mill; moreover, the baker's oven may not be working properly and may emit noxious gases into the atmosphere, which, combined with those of a van which travels short distances but is highly pollutant, is perhaps worse than long journeys by ship or by train. One is tempted to say that sustainability is relative too, but only because the example I have been considering is a hypothetical one: these data can in fact be precisely calculated and the judgment would be fairly objective.

The time has come for everybody—producers, traders, institutions, associations, and individual citizens—to ask themselves whether their lifestyle is sustainable and to take steps to make sustainability measurable and testable. That our lifestyle has not been sustainable until now is an established fact: the Millennium Ecosystem Assessment report quoted in the first chapter is quite clear on this point, and it is only the most recent and exhaustive of many reports that have been made over the past twenty years. It was in the early 1970s that the first warnings were sounded: the growth of our economy had limits which we had almost reached, and our consumption of resources far exceeded what was available in nature. The first major debate then took place in 1992, with the Rio International Conference on the Environment and Development; at the end of that meeting, the world governments drew up a document, *Agenda 21*, which was supposed to lay down the criteria of sustainability for the next decade. It was an important document, which discussed the struggle against desertification, the protection of the climate, biodiversity, and many other problems affecting the whole world. It contained all the guidelines for the effort that needed to be made by governments and individual citizens. Ten years later, at another conference in Johannesburg, it was clear that all those good intentions had not produced any concrete results. The guidance that had been given had not been followed, simply because there were no rules and sanctions, and people were completely free to decide what was sustainable or otherwise. No one can really be said to be against sustainability, but changing one's lifestyle to conform to it is a different matter. It is difficult enough to do on a personal level, let alone on a national one.

Environmental sustainability is the first and most important prerequisite for a "clean" product, and at present it remains a matter for the private judgment of the consumer, not least because it may conflict with economic practicality (and with the economic interests of the producers), as well as with questions of social justice (as we shall see later). But that is not all: environmental sustainability can be measured; it is based on precise knowledge and information that is not provided to us, and which we cannot be bothered or are not able to obtain. To strive to ensure that this information (the agricultural methods used to produce the raw materials, the areas of production, the forms of transport used, the respect for biodiversity and for ecosystems throughout the production process) be made public and accessible (ideally on the label) is the task of the new gastronome. In this case, too, it is a question of social responsibility. The responsibility for what is sustainable is shared by all of us: the farmer, the processor (whether industrial or artisanal), the politicians who can legislate about it, and the ordinary people who every day, while they are shopping, can influence production with their purchasing decisions.

The second question we must ask ourselves when we evaluate a product, after we have asked ourselves whether it is "good," must be, is it "clean," is it "sustainable"? If the information necessary for us to make a judgment is not available, let us apply pressure to ensure that is made available. We must all be able to evaluate and to choose in accordance with our evaluations; that is the only path that leads to quality.

2.2 Agriculture

The prime suspect in our investigation of environmental sustainability is agriculture. Since the 1950s, the progressive industrialization of agricultural methods has profoundly changed the nature of the countryside. The use of pesticides and chemical fertilizers has drastically increased, killing the bacterial microflora that keep the soil alive and fertile in many areas of the world. The indiscriminate exploitation of water resources to cultivate ever more productive and thirsty varieties has consumed huge reserves, and at the same time the water-bearing strata have been polluted by the fertilizers and pesticides. The desertification and drying out of the soil is occurring in places where it was unheard of a few years ago (to say that the southern Italian region of Basilicata is at risk of desertification is a very different matter from saying that sub-Saharan Africa is running the same risk, is it not?). Intensive stock farming has not only worsened the quality of our meat and led to the extinction of many excellent breeds, it also pollutes the soil with excrement that is full of antibiotics and other substances present in the fodder which are not broken down or absorbed by the animals. (Why does the treatment of sewage from an intensive stock farm have to be carefully regulated? Why can it not reenter the natural cycle in the normal way? It is only dung, after all: this is quite a paradox.)

In many parts of the world, the countryside is increasingly coming to resemble an industrial landscape: there is no life in it. Farmers are nowhere to be seen—they have become more and more like factory workers who mass-produce goods. Landscapes have been irremediably scarred; the fields express their failing struggle for survival in their faded colors, alongside ugly buildings—stalls, sheds, and gigantic machines offend the eye that surveys the place where our food is produced, but where death hangs in the air, arousing feelings that are far from bucolic.

We have gone far beyond the breaking point; we need an immediate change of direction and a profound change in mentality. Agriculture must be deindustrialized; the earth and the natural environment must be given priority again. The earth must not be allowed to die, or kept alive like a terminally ill patient, with traumatic methods. Stressed soil does not produce properly, and in the end produces only death. Stressed soil is not the result of a harmonious relationship between man and nature: it is nothing but a food-producing machine—a sad machine, which does not generate happiness.

How, then, can agriculture be deindustrialized?

We must begin, in this case too, by rejecting everything that is *unnatural*, everything that introduces *unsustainable* artifice into the relationship between man and the earth.

Pesticides and chemical fertilizers are not sustainable as a method of production. They are useful in extreme cases, but we cannot keep the earth alive in a perpetually critical condition. They must be avoided as much as possible; they are harmful to the land and to our health, and are not conducive to life in the long term. If we go on like this, we will leave our children nothing but barren fields.

Intensive methods of production, both for plants and for animals, must be rejected. We do not need to increase production. We need to improve and "clean" it. We cannot demand more each year from the soil or from a cow, or expect a chicken to grow in half the time it would naturally do: they are not machines, they are *living things*, and their natural mechanism, if it breaks down, cannot be repaired like an industrial milling-machine.

We must give preference to local varieties and breeds: their survival ensures the biodiversity that enables the natural system to regulate itself. They are part of the ecosystem where they originated and evolved, and are a guarantee of the maintenance of that ecosystem. They ensure a wider variety of tastes, and their genetic heritage is a legacy to all humankind. If they are catalogued and preserved, they can help us find solutions where none seemed to exist: in this way, modern genetic technologies can help make up for the losses, instead of impoverishing biodiversity even further. Industrial breeds and varieties created for productive purposes reduce biodiversity and require too many natural resources in order to be nourished and complete their life cycle. They are not good; they are not clean.

Genetically modified organisms (GMOs) must be rejected. I will not go into the question of whether they are harmful to human health (this has not been conclusively proved; longer-term studies are needed, because they are such a new technology); I will not dwell on the ethical considerations (to what extent is it permissible for man to interfere with living beings? Should crossbreeds be made which would not normally occur in nature?

Is it possible to patent a living thing?); nor shall I discuss whether they are economically advantageous for farmers (though the experience and data available to us after the first years of commercialization in the United States indicate total failure).

GMOs are not sustainable from the environmental point of view: more than one study has shown that their impact is often excessive, comparable at best to that of hybrids used for intensive cultivation. Some kinds of GMO (especially corn) are highly contaminant of conventional crops: they invade other fields and spread throughout the environment. GMOs are the "perfect" product of the agricultural industry, the pinnacle reached in the quest for the "perfect variety": more resistant, more productive, the ideal monoculture. But even leaving aside assessments of their environmental compatibility, which appear to be very negative but which have yet to be completely proved (though the first studies seem very clear), they are the prime product of a productive system which subverts every principle of naturalness. The system is wrong: GMOs are the highest expression of a concept of agricultural production which no longer has any *raison d'être* because it is unsustainable from every point of view.

Monoculture must be rejected. It is the embodiment of the impoverishment of biodiversity in the fields and soil. Extensive monocultures remove both the good weeds and the bad; in order to make room for themselves, they eliminate the flora and fauna native to the ecosystem into which they are introduced. Woods, hedges, beneficial insects, birds, amphibians—almost everything disappears in the face of hectares of vines, corn, and olive trees. This is true even in the case of organic farming: if the monoculture is too extensive, it threatens biodiversity.

In the case of products that are not grown or raised, but simply picked, the same principle of sustainability in the production of raw materials applies. For example, we should sound the alarm about fishing, which must be sustainable and must not irreparably exhaust reserves of fish; the state of the seas is perhaps even worse than that of the soil when it comes to pollution, the reduction of biodiversity, overfishing, and intensive exploitation for food purposes.[40]

Deindustrializing agriculture means rejecting a system. It is not just a question of introducing techniques different from the present ones such as small-scale production, organic farming, and biodynamics. Even crops that do not involve the use of chemical agents can be unsustainable if they are part of the agroindustrial system of food production—if they reflect a reductionist and profit-oriented mindset, which takes no account of the environmental costs and which has no respect for the life of the earth and of those who live on it. Deindustrializing agriculture requires a new relationship between man and nature, an approach which is more open to complexity and which draws on all the scientific tools, both modern and traditional, to evaluate the sustainability of a new model of production.

2.3 Processing

By *processing,* I mean here any kind of human intervention between the raw material and the final product, any human action concerned with processing—technical know-how, talent, tradition, or innovation. It goes without saying that in this case, too, the food production industry is another prime suspect in the investigation into the judgment of sustainability. Fueled by intensive agricultural methods, propelled by techniques that make it possible to destroy and reconstruct the natural taste and appearance of a product, and reinforced by global distribution networks, industry is responsible for another unsustainable model of food production. Let me make myself clear: I am not saying that the industrial model should be eliminated entirely, merely that it must be brought into line with sustainability. The environmental costs must be included in the balance sheets, quantified in some way, and paid for. Otherwise, there are no limits.

It is not industry itself that is unsustainable; there are examples of industries that produce good products, have an environmental policy, and are respectful of their workers. But we should always be wary of those who exploit this scrupulousness for promotional purposes, for they often conceal other far more serious unsustainabilities. It does not impress me if

Monsanto channels a small percentage of its profits into sustainable projects: almost all multinationals do so nowadays, to salve their consciences. I want *all* their productive processes to be sustainable, I want them to include everything *in the accounts*, even the costs paid by the environment and all of us who live in it. It does not impress me if a proportion of their profits is donated to charitable causes in partial compensation of the damage they have caused; that damage should not be done in the first place and should never have to be paid for later.

But let us not put all the blame on industry (although it deserves a great deal of it, given the scale of its production and the constant stream of unsustainable inventions it churns out): let us reject its model, but admit, for the sake of intellectual honesty, that many other activities which at first sight seem more harmless are in fact equally harmful. Man's hand must always be light in processing raw materials: just as he should respect the original tastes, so he should respect the environment.

In this vein, I should point out the crucial importance of the choices made by small processors, particularly those who enjoy the greatest prestige and the greatest media exposure: the chefs. It is up to them to promote sustainable agriculture, to create virtuous production cycles, and to seek out farmers and artisans (from as close at hand as possible) who use sustainable methods in their work. Cooking, as a body of noble and scientific knowledge, has a duty to reject anything that is not produced in accordance with nature. Such products are not in the interests of good cuisine, and cooks who strive to serve good food, competing to be the best, know this perfectly well. Let them say it loud and clear, then: let them indicate the provenance of their products in their menus, let them recommend the best agricultural and artisanal goods. Let them make their own quest for excellence the driving force behind sustainable development at all levels, including the home.

Where processing is concerned, we are, again, all partly to blame: we are implicated each time we buy a product that does not respect the environment in its various phases of production. So we must do our best to ensure that we are aware of the methods of processing, and we must demand the necessary information. Let the consumer who is tempted by a very low price ask what makes that price possible. How many public subsidies were given in order to make the product so cheap? How much damage was done to the environment and to biodiversity by the intensive agriculture that produced it for the food industry? How much pollution did those who produced it generate through their production methods and through the use of artificial agents in a process that ought to be always in harmony with nature?

2.4 Transport

For a food to be "clean," it is not just the phases of agriculture and processing that must be sustainable; there are often other factors that we do not consider because we take them for granted, but environmental costs lie hidden everywhere. Food produced and consumed locally, for example, can actually be more sustainable, "greener," than organic food produced further away. This was the provocative conclusion reached by professors Tim Lang, of London University, and Jules Pretty, of the University of Essex, in a highly interesting study recently published in the *Food Policy Journal.*[41]

The authors set out to calculate scientifically the costs of the so-called *food miles*, the distance that food travels before it reaches our tables: they came to the conclusion that if the British restricted their consumption to food produced within a twenty-kilometer radius of their homes, the total annual savings for the country would be £2.1 billion. On the basis of a typical household budget, they succeeded in calculating the cost in millions of pounds of the pollution caused by pesticides, exhaust emissions into the atmosphere, soil erosion, the reduction of biodiversity, and the various effects on human health. Then, using official British statistics, they calculated the cost (in pence per kilometer by each means of transport) of each journey from the farm to the supermarket and from the supermarket to the home. They meticulously took into account all the various forms of transport, even noting the differences between a home delivery, a shopping expedition by bike or on foot, and one made by car. The results are surprising. Totaling up the pollution produced by intensive agricultural methods, the various journeys the food has to make, and the subsidies paid to agriculture, the hidden costs are equivalent to 11.8 percent of the price paid by the consumer on a typical shopping basket full of conventional British agricultural produce. And these costs of course devolve upon the community.

There had been few attempts to make this kind of calculation before now; people often talk about environmental costs, but this is perhaps the first time that they have been quantified so precisely. The authors' provocative suggestion is that if the British consumed only conventional foods that were locally produced and went shopping either by bicycle or on foot, the hidden costs would be about 7 percent—exactly the same as if they consumed only organic food produced on the continent of Europe and went shopping by car.

Whatever the merits of this suggestion, which certainly makes for good headlines—the ideal, of course, would be food that is local *and* organic—it cannot be denied that the two scholars have identified an effect of the producer's location which had been previously underestimated. The original purpose of their study was to discover all the hidden ecological costs of food production; instead, they discovered these statistics for *food miles*, which even they themselves had not foreseen.

The choices that consumers make between organic and conventional and between local and global have very important repercussions on the environment and on agricultural systems: I repeat, these are quantifiable data that must be treated as real costs.

Wider publicizing of the statistics concerning food miles would certainly influence consumer behavior, and labeling should be a step further in this direction. Nowadays, it is compulsory to indicate the place of origin of fruit, vegetables, fish, and meat, but in many cases the indications are still too generic. Besides, in the case of many processed foods it is almost impossible to trace the origin of the raw materials. If everything were clearly stated on the label, and if consumers were educated to be aware of the cost of transporting food, I am sure that a gradual relocalization of production systems would not be long in coming.

Nor would it be a bad idea to suggest that governments develop an appropriate policy of taxation, incentives, and regulatory mechanisms. To include the price in food miles on the label (alongside a description of the method of production and a more detailed list of ingredients, which removed all possibility of misinterpretation, for example in the case of flavorings) would be an excellent marketing ploy, as well as a service to the community, who want to be able to exercise their spending power by choosing food that is as clean and local as possible.

2.5 Limits: clean as an objective

I have tried to give a brief survey of the main aspects of environmental sustainability (social sustainability still remains to be considered): I cannot make any claim to exhaustiveness, given the complexity of the subject, but I have attempted to draw attention to the meaning of "sustainable" and to give an overview of the areas in which evaluations need to be made.

It is difficult to achieve absolute objectivity, but the data available in this case is considerably more factual than it was in the case of "good," and less related to purely cultural factors. How can we orient ourselves amid this mass of information? In the first place, we can use our common sense, on the basis of the "educated" awareness that was mentioned earlier. It should also be pointed out that common sense is dictated primarily by our awareness of *limits*—limits which we must know how to handle, and beyond which there is no growth and no development, but only destructive growth, long-term economic loss, ecological loss, and cultural impoverishment.

There are limits of production: a vegetable, a breed, a place, and an ecosystem have structural limits that we cannot exceed without altering their characteristics. For example Colonnata *lardo* (a kind of fatty bacon) can only be made in the town of Colonnata, in Tuscany, because of the microclimate that exists there, and one cannot expect to fill the whole area with the well-known marble basins in which it is matured. There is a limit to the amount of *lardo* these basins can take; to make them too big would be to *alter the nature of the product*. There is also a structural limit, which cannot be exceeded merely to satisfy the demand for Colonnata *lardo*: one ought to aim rather at differentiation and at the production of different kinds of *lardo* in other places, using similar methods and giving them different names.

Consider that some native cows produce tiny amounts of milk compared to Holstein cows, which are veritable milk machines. But the milk of these native cows has unique characteristics and should not be replaced simply for the sake of increasing productivity. Nor can one increase indefinitely the number of native cows, which may well be accustomed (and physically suited, by constitution) to grazing rather than to other kinds of farming.

The Langhe, in Piedmont, an area mainly used for the production of great wines, should not become a vine monoculture simply because the wines are very successful on the international market. In the areas where Barolo is produced, we should not try to plant vines everywhere, even on north-facing hills (the worst position for a vineyard; in days gone by, no one would have ever dreamed of doing such a thing), relying on fertilizers and chemical pesticides to make the vines grow despite the conditions. The soil is destroyed and dried out; woods, fields, pastures and hedges, with all their flora and fauna, are removed to make room for the vineyards. Biodiversity is diminished, and the ecosystem of the hills is reduced to being a winemaking machine: this indiscriminate exploitation will soon seriously affect the production of the great wines in the region. The limit is being exceeded.

A distributor of food products should not transport products indiscriminately from one side of the world to the other merely for his own convenience. Food mile pollution would increase and serious imbalances might result.

There is a limit to abundance. World food production is already sufficient to feed us all—why should we increase it? Where is the need for inventing GMOs? Why do we persist in exceeding the limits of the earth? All we achieve by this is the creation of new limits, until it is impossible to rectify the situation. As the poet Giuseppe Ungaretti wrote:

> Man, monotonous universe,
> thinks he is increasing his goods,
> but the only numberless things produced
> by his frantic hands are limits

Managing limits is the first step toward sustainability, and not just in an environmental sense. But in order to achieve this, we must renounce economic growth as the sole criterion of human progress. We calculate our fortunes—the fortunes of a state—on the basis of its GNP (gross national product). I agree with the proposal of Amartya Sen, the Indian Nobel Prize winner for economics and an expert in the economics of happiness: we need to start calculating our GNH, gross national happiness. Let us ask ourselves which limits we have already exceeded and which ones we are about to exceed: let us learn to change our ways and to manage them. Within the limits, we can find all the growth opportunities we want, provided that we do not count money alone. Within the limits, there is the "good," indeed all the "goods" of the world; within the limits, there is the "clean," there is *quality*.

2.6 Is clean good?

Clean, sustainable production creates all the right conditions for the good. It is important to add this latter consideration, because in any discussion of quality it is a fundamental concept. Soils that are not stressed, cheapened, and killed by unnatural substances bear better fruit. Animals raised in a natural way, without haste and without exceeding the structural limits of an activity such as stock farming, can produce meat and milk (and hence also cheese) with sensory characteristics far superior to those of animals that have been exploited, "drugged," and kept in miserable conditions in small stalls without any regard for their well-being.

Finally, a product that does not make long journeys will be fresher and will preserve its gustatory potential better. Chef Alain Ducasse once said to me in an interview: "If I pay a lot for a mullet in Paris, it probably comes from Dakar. It doesn't make economic sense; its journey has created pollution and it is tired after the journey. It cannot be better than a mullet caught on the northern coast of France and brought to the market the same morning."

The clean creates the conditions for the good. However, the equation "clean equals good" is not valid. A good product is not necessarily clean; the fishing of date mussels has been banned for years because it destroys kilometers of rocky coast in order to catch a product which is so slow-growing that it cannot guarantee the survival of the species—though they are delicious. And a clean product, even if it has all the right prerequisites to be good, can become very bad in the hands of unskilled producers. There are some products of organic agriculture, for example, which are totally unacceptable from the point of view of taste. We cannot stake everything on the added value of a product which does not harm the environment; we must also work for the good.

However, it should be repeated that a clean product is of the greatest significance to taste; the probability that the two values, clean and good, will go hand in hand and be causally linked is very high.

2.7 Is it clean?

The second of the three essential and interdependent prerequisites for a quality product is that it be *clean*—clean for the earth and for the ecosystems. Clean is sustainable; it does not pollute, it does nothing to put the earth in a condition of ecological deficit. Sustainability is obtained by respecting a criterion of naturalness, and by being aware of limits, whether human, vegetable, animal, or productive. The new gastronome's task is to be aware of these limits, to learn how to recognize them: to produce, or support the production of, foods that are sustainable throughout their journey from the field to the table.

This is a commitment to knowledge and requires study and access to accurate information about what we eat. This, too, is a political task, whose purpose is to improve the quality of life, and the clean itself improves the quality of life. Should anyone dismiss the idea that unsustainable production is harmful to the land, and continue to produce and consume in a manner incompatible with our happiness (and therefore continue to produce unhappiness), I say that the clean has become indispensable. The earth is dying, with ever-increasing rapidity.

Clean is respect for others and for ourselves; to work to ensure that it is practiced by everyone is another part of our civilizing mission. This is a concern of the gastronome, and leads to the eco-gastronome, who enjoys, knows, and eats in the awareness that he must leave a better planet to future generations.

{**DIARY 10**} GREEN CALIFORNIA

In autumn 2003, I participated in a conference at the University of Berkeley, California, attended by hundreds of students, professors, and farmers. I was in very good company: Vandana Shiva; Wendell Berry, the farmer poet from Kentucky; Michael Pollan, of the Graduate School of Journalism at Berkeley; and Alice Waters, perhaps the most distinguished chef in the United States. My stay in California lasted about a week, and during that period I took the opportunity to find out more about the powerful local organic farming sector, and to interview one of the founding fathers of agroecological theory, Professor Miguel Altieri (see pp. 67–68).

For once I neglected my contacts with the Californian wine world, which were what first took me there in the early 1980s, and concentrated instead on the wonderful results achieved by a largely reconverted agricultural sector which produced excellent raw materials without recourse to fertilizers and artificial manure. I was very curious to find out how far they had got, and to talk to the farmers who were leading this minor revolution that ran counter to current trends elsewhere in the world.

By coincidence, the program of my trip included in one day a visit to the luxurious and very important Ferry Plaza farmers' market and an afternoon at the university talking to Altieri. What follows is a diary of that day.

Morning. The cool morning began quite early: if you are going to the market, it is best to be ready by seven o'clock at the latest. The sun was not yet warm enough when, in the company of my chef friend Alice Waters, I entered an elegantly refurbished area of the docks; pretty little coffee shops were serving warm mugs of excellent organic fair-trade coffee; sumptuous bakeries were putting out all sorts of good things, spreading the fragrant aroma of some wonderful kinds of bread. Oil and wine producers were offering samples in marquees, while hundreds of open-air stalls were selling excellent products: fruit and vegetables, fish, meat, sausages, and even flowers—fresh, healthy-looking food, all carefully marked *organic*.

One could have easily spent a fortune there. The prices were astronomical, twice or even three times as high as those of "conventional" products. But how hard it is to produce things so well, and what costs are involved in obtaining certification! I am convinced that the farmers' intelligent, productive efforts deserve to be paid for generously, so I was not too scandalized by the prices, even though they were those of a boutique. Yes, a boutique: for I soon realized I was in an extremely exclusive place (bear in mind that this is one of the oldest and most important farmers' markets in town, *la crème de la crème*). The amiable ex-hippies and young dropouts-turned-farmers greeted their customers with a smile and offered generous samples of their products to a clientele whose social status was pretty clear: either wealthy or very wealthy.

Alice Waters introduced me to dozens of farmers: they were all well-to-do college graduates, former employees of Silicon Valley, many of them young. Meanwhile, their customers, most of whom seemed to be actresses, went home clutching their peppers, squashes, and apples, showing them off like jewels, status symbols.

Two of the producers in particular struck me: a young man with a long beard and a man who was selling oil. The former, with long hair and a plaid flannel shirt, held his lovely little blond-haired daughter in his arms and told me, in a conspiratorial tone, that he had to drive two hundred miles to come and sell in that market: he charged incredibly high prices for his squashes, it was "a cinch," and in just two monthly visits he could earn more than enough to maintain his family and spend hours surfing on the beach.

The latter, who wore a tie, extolled the beauties of his farm: it consisted of hundreds of hectares of olive trees, stretching as far as the eye could see, and nothing else. While I was tasting his excellent organic oil on a slice of bread which reminded me of Tuscan bread—absolutely delicious—I was thinking of what he must have uprooted and cleared away in order to grow all those plants, each one of them impeccably *organic*.

Afternoon. In the early afternoon, with those odors and aromas and the faces of the marvelous farmers' market still in my head, I was sweating in a taxi (it lacked the usually ubiquitous American air-conditioning) on the way to Berkeley for my appointment with Miguel Altieri. The professor, an entomologist, teaches agroecology at the university. He spends six months a year in California and the other six elsewhere in the world, especially in South America, where he carries out fieldwork and projects of sustainable, family-based, organic farming. He is a champion of biodiversity, with his theory that agricultural systems, like all ecosystems, ought to have all the necessary capacities for self-regulation, without the intervention of external factors such as pesticides and fertilizers.

According to Altieri, the existing biodiversity—on which farmers' knowledge has been molded for thousands of years—and local people's know-how are the only basis for developing agricultural systems that are sufficiently productive and respectful of cultural diversity all around the world. By blending the local farmers' knowledge with the discoveries of "mainstream" science, it is possible to create a clean and productive agriculture which will foster human well-being while respecting nature.

I walked across the beautiful Berkeley campus under a warm, dazzling sun (green California gets it even in the fall) and reached Altieri's small office. I listened spellbound for over an hour to his theories, conversing in Spanish (he is Chilean) and relishing his militant passion and the unmistakable honesty of this man who works and struggles for a better world. Biodiversity before all else: this is the only secret behind sustainable development. His aversion to the use of chemical substances in agriculture is clear, absolute, and motivated. He proposes alternative methods with such utter conviction that in South America he is considered a luminary and is respected by universities, research centers, NGOs, and governments.

In his opinion, the main task is "to promote sustainable agriculture; a development program which is socially equitable, environmentally healthy, economically affordable, and culturally sensitive."[42]

I asked him what he thought of organic farming and its rapid expansion in California, wanting to test his agroecological "extremism." He replied:

> There are many cases of organic farming that are not sustainable, because they create a vast monoculture, one that relies on the use of integrated pesticides which greatly reduce the surrounding biodiversity: vast stretches of vineyards in Chile and in Italy, huge planta-

tions of vegetables in California, hectares and hectares of olive groves in Spain.[43]

Olive groves . . . I thought of the man I had met that morning. I remembered the faces of my wine-producer friends in southern Piedmont, who, since Barolo sells well, have in the space of a few years planted vines everywhere, even in ditches, removing woodland and fields, indeed most of the surrounding biodiversity.

Altieri continued:

And in addition to the environmental question, there is also a socioeconomic one: nowadays in California there is a lot of organic agriculture which is unsustainable because, although it has a limited environmental impact, it exists at the expense of people who are paid very little, just as in conventional agriculture. Hosts of Mexican immigrants exploited like slaves, with no rights and earning a pittance. It is not fair, because the organic product is sold at a much higher price than the product of conventional farming. And only the very rich can afford it, the fruits of this work; the minorities don't eat organic food in the United States.[44]

I had seen confirmation of this a few hours earlier, and indeed, as Altieri flowed on:

In California, 2 percent of organic producers make 50 percent of the total amount produced by the industry in this sector; I use the term "industry" advisedly: we are facing the same problems as conventional agriculture. The concentration of production, the exploitation of the work of ethnic minorities, monocultures, the reduction of biodiversity, and prices determined by a free market which is not sustainable. Social sustainability can be achieved through public intervention, through politics: in Brazil, in those regions where the Workers' Party controls the local government, all food served in public cafeterias must by law be organic and must be produced by small local producers at fair but accessible prices. Agroecology has a scientific basis, but it also has profound political implications, because it is badly in need of public intervention: before an agroecological approach can be established in Latin America, there must be agrarian reform and public intervention in the market to protect small farmers or to guarantee fair prices for producers and consumers. All these factors are crucial, and they affect both science and politics.[45]

Evening. On my way back to town, I pondered those words and the market I had visited. Organic farming is undoubtedly a very good thing; it is an excellent alternative to agroindustry, and I do not like to find fault with people—my friends of that morning—who sell products that are so naturally good. But perhaps it is better to have doubts. Reality is complex and resists labels. There is a risk that technocratic thought, when it is deeply rooted, may shape and influence even those tendencies that are opposed to the system, thereby creating other anomalies.

As the outskirts of town flashed by outside the window of the taxi, chains of fast-food joints succeeded one another on almost every block. They were all crowded with ordinary people, very different people from the customers I had seen at the farmers' market.

In the evening I returned to Berkeley, and went to Chez Panisse, the restaurant owned by my friend Alice Waters, where I had a memorable dinner based on raw materials so fresh you could almost taste the life that had animated the vegetables only a few hours earlier. They served me the best *agnolotti* I have ever eaten. At Berkeley! Green California... *vive la contradiction!*

....

3. FAIR

The third and last prerequisite for a quality product is that it should be *fair*. In food production, the word "fair" connotes social justice, respect for workers and their know-how, rurality and the country life, pay adequate to work, gratification in producing well, and the definitive revaluation of the small farmer, whose historical position in society has always been last.

It is not acceptable that those who produce our food, those people (half the total world population) who work to grow crops, raise livestock, and turn nature into food, should be treated like social outcasts and struggle to make ends meet amid all kinds of difficulty. In different parts of the world, farmers are facing a vast range of problems: history has given them a different relationship with the countryside, but few farmers prosper (and of those lucky few, most are neither "clean" nor "good" and do not produce quality food). The global food system should be engaged in finding out what is fair for everybody, in accordance with the characteristics of the various geographical areas of the world, but at present it is only creating unfairness and terrible hardship.

Our definition of "fair" is closely linked with the crucial concepts of social and economic *sustainability*, the dependants of ecological sustainability, the missing elements in our descriptions of sustainability in the broadest sense of the term. The fair, socially speaking, means fairness for the people who work the soil, respect for those who still love it and treat it with respect, as a source of life. *La tera l'e' basa*, "the land is low," they say in Piedmont: the farmer's life is a hard one, and the conditions to which many of them have been reduced cry out for revenge. Agribusiness has turned small farmers into factory workers, slaves, paupers with no hopes for the future. Millions of farmers in the world do not even own the land they work.

We must create a new system that will give these people due recognition for the vital role they play: we cannot do without the farmers, the *producing communities*. It is on this concept of "community," of destiny and belonging to the human race, that the new system must be founded. Starting from them, from these producing communities, we must build a worldwide net-work that is capable of opposing the dominant system. We must put man, the land, and food back in the center: a *human* food network which, in harmony with nature and respectful of all diversity, will promote quality: good, clean, and fair.

3.1 Social sustainability

From a social point of view, "sustainable" means promoting quality of life through dignified jobs that guarantee sustenance and fair remuneration. It means guaranteeing equity and democracy all over the world, giving everyone the right to choose their future. There are still too many peasants, farm laborers, that are virtual slaves who work to produce food and cannot live above the poverty line in a world that can produce enough for everybody.

In Latin America, the big *fazendeiros* exploit the work of farm laborers, giving them no rights and paying them so little as to effectively reduce them to slavery. In Africa, farmers are dying of hunger; Indian peasants commit suicide, crushed by the com-petition of agribusiness. Agricultural production in many parts of the world is indistinguishable from industrial production before the advent of the trade unions. Peasants die on the job or leave the country to go to live in miserable conditions in huge cities like Mexico City, Lima, Saô Paulo, New Delhi, and Beijing. At the same time, farmers in the rich areas of the world who want to produce the "good" and the "clean" find it difficult to compete with the low prices, supported by subsidies, which agroindustry can afford. The system is perverse: it does not allow other mod-els, but where will this all end? Who will produce our food?

The small farmer can save the world from the abyss: let us give him the chance to do so.

We must create the conditions for a new, rebalanced global order based on social justice for those who work the land, for the real and potential custodians of our land. In the areas that have been conquered by agribusiness, we must give small producers back their dignity and encourage "clean" small-scale production.

But in order to make this possible, those who exceed the limits will have to be penalized, and governments must support the birth—the rebirth—of a *new rurality*. By this I mean a countryside that is "clean" and attractive, and not only in the aesthetic sense of the word: a pleasant place to live where the quality of life is guaranteed. At present, wherever agribusiness triumphs, the countryside is a lifeless place, lacking in basic amenities (small businesses, meeting points, places where one can enjoy the beauties of nature), and often ugly. Its main function is that of a dormitory for city workers attracted by a nostalgia (which remains unsatisfied) for the country life and the fact that real estate prices are lower (not surprisingly, since there is no public transport, and everyone travels by car, congesting the city centers and making the air unbreathable). A new rurality in the rich areas: this is another prime objective.

In other parts of the world, where conditions are often extremely serious, pressure must be put, first of all, on organizations such as the World Trade Organization or the World Bank, which have not only heightened the problems of inequality with their commercial and economic regulations, but do their utmost to maintain the status quo. The situation is full of terrible inequalities, and I am certainly not the first person to have decried it. Secondly, we must ensure that governments, overburdened as they are with debts, begin to work seriously to achieve lasting development, and will not be influenced by the agribusiness lobby, which is always making grand promises but is only interested in expanding its own market. We need international controls on the levels of corruption in certain governments, which exploit humanitarian aid to enrich themselves and contribute to the destruction of the weak domestic markets; the latter are weakened by the flood of free agricultural produce, and the collapse of the meager local production is the inevitable result. We should be providing incentives to this local production, in accordance with tradition, primarily in the interests of self-sufficiency, giving all peoples sovereignty over their own food supplies; people must be able to produce *their own* food by themselves.

Restoring the balance of a whole world is one of the hardest tasks imaginable, but the means by which a change of course can be made without renouncing the search for quality should be clear by now: small-scale production, self-sufficiency, crop diversification, the revival and use of traditional methods, full respect for a fruitful interaction with the local biodiversity, and agroecology.

3.2 *Economic sustainability*

In addition to the social point of view, in the context of "fairness" there is also an economic sustainability which needs to be assessed. I have already mentioned fair remuneration for farmers. It is not possible for one liter of olive oil to cost less than seven or eight dollars: if that does happen, it can only mean that the farmer is not being paid a fair amount, that production costs are higher than the final price, and that somewhere along the food production line unfairness must have occurred. It is not fair that the illegal Mexican immigrants who work in California should be paid a pittance. It is not fair that Indian peasants, who find it difficult to produce their own vegetables, should have to cope with unfair competition from subsidized Western products or from surpluses created by market dumping.

The *fair-trade* market from this point of view is doing a very good job; it has introduced a different approach to the food economy and should therefore be encouraged and respected, though in my view it ought to be combined with structural interventions in the producing communities and not just limited to the fixing of a fair price. Fair trade must never forget the other two aspects of quality: clean and good. Sometimes it does, and this is the worst advertisement it could give itself in its struggle to rectify the unfair conventions of the market.

But there is also another economic aspect, which brings us back to social justice. The global financial world, the battleground of multinationals and unfair trade, has made money an elusive and immaterial entity. Capital is not "patient"; people do not invest in businesses which guarantee social justice and the redemption of peasants, or which have a low environmental impact. A movement of money on the stock exchange can seal the fate of tens of thousands of small farmers at a stroke. We need a *slower*, more "patient" investment policy, which operates outside the classical framework of finance: sustainable models of investment for the agricultural communities, which give them time to grow without expecting immediate profits. Slowing down economics means bringing it down to earth, for the earth. The World Bank, the leading international financial organization, should take note of these problems and act accordingly. The imposition of a Western free-market financial-economic model in countries that are structurally very different from ours has only served to burden them with crippling debts, squeezing them in a vice from which they cannot extricate themselves.[46]

Money must be brought back down to earth, it must be made available to the young who want to go and cultivate the land, so as to stimulate the vitality of the countryside and restore the balance of wealth in the world, in a line that runs from the smallest farmer to the largest capital transfers.

3.3 *The land for those who cultivate it*

The idea of a return to the land presupposes that there is a real possibility of achieving it. In many parts of the world, farmers abandon the land and sell it off to landowners who practice extensive agriculture; those who hold out are besieged by the chemical pollution that "modern" methods pour into the environment around their small properties. In many countries, farmers are still waiting for agrarian reform which will make uncultivated lands available to them (as in Brazil, for example, where the movement of the Sem Terra, "the landless ones," has two million members) and create conditions in which they can cultivate their smallholdings without being crushed by the power of agribusiness. Even in the rich areas of the world, many people find it difficult to go back to the land: young people cannot raise the money to buy land, and farmers often work on rented land on behalf of big companies, so they are unable to exert any long-term influence by practicing good, clean, and fair small-scale agriculture.

The problem of land ownership is still serious around the world, and seeking out "fair" products also means rejecting those that are the result of productive systems which create this regrettable situation: for often those who cultivate the land cannot own it, and are not free to choose the kind of agriculture they favor.

3.4 Always "the last wheel of the cart"

There is an Italian expression which aptly describes the condition of farmers throughout history: they always have been, and continue to be, *l'ultima ruota del carro*, "the last wheel of the cart," the lowest sector of society. They have worked either for landowners—as in the feudal system with its hierarchical scale, where the military and the clergy were at the top and the peasants who worked for the sustenance of all were at the bottom—or for political leaders. They have always worked for an elite that did not want to dirty its hands producing food. Whether or not they owned land, their condition has been one of subordination: the means of dominion have changed with the historical periods and the cultural contexts, but the rule of the last wheel of the cart has prevailed. Even today, the situation in which farmers find themselves is not very different. If we consider the world as a whole, this subordination manifests itself in different ways from one macro-area to another. Progress has changed the styles and techniques of "dominion," but those who produce food, those who feed humanity, are always at the bottom of the social scale.

We must, of course, distinguish between two large groups: the rich, schizophrenic West, and the developing countries, which are at the mercy of the momentous upheavals that we are currently experiencing.

The "schizophrenic" situation in that part of the world which has solved its own food-supply problems derives from a very particular dualism, now that class divisions have diminished almost to the point of disappearing. On the one hand, we have a few rich farmers, committed to the agroindustrial model of production, who produce vast quantities of mediocre food for people who are poor, or at least not rich. On the other hand, we have a few small farmers who struggle to produce high-quality goods and who find it impossible (except in the case of the most exclusive status symbols, such as certain wine productions) to live a dignified life, such is the pressure of the competition. The latter produce food for a rich elite, who can afford the fruits of their labor, which are sometimes distributed thousands of kilometers away. As far as social justice is concerned, in the rich West the situation is complex: is it fair to harm the interests of those farmers who have made money through massive and extensive production in favor of small farmers who produce quality food? In reality, however, this part of the world seems to be balancing out; we have already seen how every tendency always produces an opposite one and how globalization has had the paradoxical effect of reviving interest in diversity and local productions. It seems that this dualism is gradually diminishing, thus making room for choices based on merit: our family food budget has significantly decreased, which means there is now a portion of our income left over that can be used to support quality products. The range of choice is expanding, and in this context anyone who acquires food products, in full awareness of the three criteria for quality, is in a good position to bring about a change. Even subsidizing policies, which are the main source of survival for the agroindustrial system, are gradually beginning to turn toward quality, as is shown by the first tentative European steps toward a reform of the Common Agricultural Policy (CAP). Consumers' persistence in choosing good, clean, and fair products can have its effect, and it will be the task of the new gastronome to draw attention to this behavior in the act of purchasing—to foster knowledge, so that the system can recover its balance and return within its limits.

However, the Western world must take into account the rest of the planet: above all, we should not expect to be able to dump the surplus of our model (which does not work anymore) in the so-called developing countries. This is not sustainable from any point of view. The developing countries must find their own way, by seeking a *food sovereignty* of their own. The most we can do is to help them and avoid looking at the problem from the Eurocentric standpoint of *conquistadores* who "discovered" America.

The developing countries, though united by the immense problems and injustices that affect them, show different levels of development in the agriculture of different areas. Africa first suffered the invasion of colonialism and was then almost left to itself and to its internal conflicts. African colonizers did not consider local gastronomies worthy of respect: they simply cancelled them out along with a form of farming which, though very basic, would have been perfectly capable of evolving of its own accord if it had been properly supported and not impeded. In other parts of the world, colonization from the agro-gastronomical point of view was less destructive and created syncretisms (such as Pan-American syncretism or that between America and Europe), which preserved part of the local agricultural cultures. But soon the agro-industrial model appeared and rapidly developing countries such as Brazil, India, and Mexico are paying the price in the form of stark polarization of the classes and areas of grinding poverty.

We find a different situation again in the Far East, especially in China. China seems to be the great threat to the Western world with its incessant economic growth, but we should consider the problem (whether real or imagined) from the point of view of social justice. In China, workers' rights are not respected. The level of pollution, along with the indiscriminate use of GMOs and of agricultural practices so noxious that they are banned in every other part of the world, show an aspect of Chinese development that few seem to take into consideration—the same problems that we used to have in the West, except that in China they are happening now and far more quickly.[47] The harm that is being done in China in the name of development is incalculable, and the system, though nominally communist, is in fact the embodiment of perfect capitalism: political homogeneity, uncontrolled exploitation of labor, and exploitation of the natural environment with no thought of the future. We need to promote a strong international reaction, not by increasing existing tariffs or imposing new ones, not by seeking complicity, but rather by rejecting such an unfair system, and making the Chinese respect the environment and their workers. If we do not, the "Chinese threat" may become huge—not because it will deprive us of wealth, but because it will drive us even more quickly toward the precipice.

Social justice, linked with the good and the clean, must become the method of development, the only one possible. These three criteria of quality will combine differently in different parts of the world, but they remain the three cardinal points on which we must build, little by little, with new tools and with the *neo-gastronomic* attitude, a new model of growth on this planet.

3.5 *Is it fair?*

The third of the three essential and interdependent prerequisites for a quality product is that it be *fair*—fair for man and for society. "Fair" is sustainable; it creates wealth, and establishes a more equitable order among the peoples of the world. Justice is obtained by respecting man—the farmer, the craftsman—and his work. It is the new gastronome's task to assess the living conditions of millions of small farmers all over the world (but particularly those close to his home), to get to know those farmers, to support the production of the "clean" and "good" ones, guaranteeing them fair remuneration through "fair trade" prices in the most serious cases.

Should anyone be tempted to ignore the complexity of the world and consume their food irresponsibly and unfairly, indifferent to social justice, I say that the fair has become indispensable. The human elite must be made up of those who produce food, not by those who consume it by consuming the land.

Fair is respect for others; working to ensure that it is pursued by everyone is another part of our civilizing mission. This is the gastronome's concern, and it leads directly to the new gastronome, who enjoys, knows, and eats in the awareness that he must leave a better earth to future generations.

CHAPTER IV

THREE IDEAS TO PUT INTO PRACTICE

The meeting room of the Hotel Marriott in 1991 was a
truly remarkable sight. We were in the heart of New York,
in Times Square, with a thousand people diligently seated,
tasting different vintages of Barbaresco; on the stage were
the legendary producer Angelo Gaja and the editor of the
magazine *Wine Spectator*. They were explaining the characteristics of Piedmont (one American asked the memorable question: "Alba is near Florence, isn't it?"—the
American concept of space is rather different from that of
the Italians), of the vines, and of the techniques of winemaking. This round table on Piedmontese wine was immediately translated into a comparative tasting guided by the
speakers, where every participant could personally experience the nuances of the various products.

All this happened in an attentive and respectful audi-
torium, as if we were at university and some luminary were
holding forth. I was struck by that visual impression, and I
understood that the operation was something more than
mere enological marketing; it was a collective cognitive
moment, of great cultural significance. It was the first time
I had attended a lecture that combined gustatory-olfactory
sensitivity with information about production methods,
and I became convinced that this operation not only could
be replicated in Italy and elsewhere in the world with
respect to wine—which occupies the most prestigious
place in gastronomy—but that it could become a model
applicable to other food products. Why not hold such discussions and comparative tastings for cheese, charcuterie,
the specialties of a particular chef, fish, or fruit, taking as
interlocutors the true repositories of experience and
knowledge about the products, namely the producers, the
farmers, the fishermen, and the craftsmen?

The formula was codified, experiments were made,
and it was officially applied for the first time by Slow Food

in 1994 during Vinitaly in Verona, the principal Italian wine fair. Slow Food participates in the Veronese event every year and always tries to bring along new ideas and to animate "gastronomically" the spaces that it occupies. That year there was a section of the fair called Grand Menu, which was our first major project, in the attention we paid not only to wine and restaurants, but also to the rest of the world of food production. Grand Menu was a microcosm of what later became the Salone del Gusto, the largest food-and-wine show in the world, which is now held every two years by Slow Food and the Regional Council of Piedmont.

On that occasion, we launched what we called the Laboratori del Gusto (Taste Workshops), which were to become one of the most expressive and significant forms of our entire movement.

Even today, when I think that at every edition of the Salone del Gusto more than thirty thousand people participate in an average of two hundred to three hundred Taste Workshops with the same attentiveness and respect that I encountered for the first time in New York, I can hardly believe it. This is in my view one of the greatest contributions that Slow Food has made to education in gastronomy, food, and taste, revolutionizing the lecturers' way of expressing themselves (including their language), identifying the best of them among the producers themselves, and bringing comparative tasting to a level which may be described as scientific, even though, given the lively, playful manner in which it is done, it seems to have very little in common with pure science. It is a method that provides the participant with some interpretative keys and makes no claims to fixing objective standards.

It is a kind of education that has entered so profoundly into Slow Food's mode of operation that it has also influenced the design of the curriculum of the University of Gastronomic Sciences (in Pollenzo, Italy). With time, the method has been enriched by another novelty, the dimension of travel, for it makes more sense to hold many of these workshops in the real places where the products originate.

And it all began in that packed meeting room of the Marriott Hotel just over fifteen years ago.

....

1. EDUCATION

The gastronome makes *knowledge* his watchword—a complex, multidisciplinary knowledge which involves the senses and the intellect, which embraces all cultures and is open and peaceable yet determined to demand transparency for reality. Good, clean, and fair are the cornerstones of this knowledge, ideas which require a great cognitive effort, the sharing of a large mass of information, and which demand that the gastronome change his approach to food—first and foremost that he restore centrality to food, equipping himself with all the tools necessary to proclaim that all human beings have a right to their *own* food, to their own choices, in harmony with their culture and with the natural environment in which they live.

The gastronome's aim, ultimately, is pleasure, happiness. This is a conscious pleasure which is not limited to pure enjoyment, but which is fortified by knowledge and is ready to be communicated, described, and shared at the table.

At present, however, the gastronome's knowledge is also the main obstacle to happiness; for, together with pleasure (with *taste*), it is denied, not communicated. It is derided or considered a superfluous exercise.

The gastronome finds himself in a minority. He must try to obtain knowledge where he can, and as he can. It might be from small-scale farmers, particularly if he can find farmers who are willing to talk about themselves. It might be from friends who share his natural passion for the good, clean, and fair. It might be from chefs, for they are the highest expression of gastronomic culture. It might be from craftsmen and all those who process food in all possible ways, or even from specialists in the various scientific disciplines related to gastronomy, presuming they also possess the sensibility of a gastronome.

This learning process, supported by the desire to keep one's senses awake, aware, and well-trained, is left to the inventiveness, the passion, the willpower, and the economic possibilities of the individual gastronome. It is not taught at school; there are no comprehensive courses. You are reduced to collecting scraps of knowledge wherever you can find them; you try to put them together according to the powers of your intelligence, and rely on exchanging ideas with others, in a continual process of personal research.

The gastronome, until today, has been of necessity self-taught; it is he who decides where, how, when, and with whom to study. His knowledge is the consequence of a precise desire, driven by the most diverse aspirations—not always those considered among the most noble by the world of culture. It is no rare occurrence for someone to arrive at a certain degree of gastronomic awareness having started from the simple—and primal—desire to *enjoy* food more, a desire which, though it attracts all the usual prejudices, is natural, just as the drive toward knowledge is normal.

The awareness of the complexity of the food system is acquired by education, study, and the exercise of the senses. So the legitimate wish to seek pleasure should never be censured, belittled, repressed, or relegated to other fields; the search for pleasure needs to be *educated*.

This is the challenge of the new gastronomy. Systems of life-long education are needed, for all ages and all people: for children, who have the right to learn how to use their senses, how food is produced and where it comes from; for parents and teachers, who are no longer able to provide a culinary education; for "consumers"—and we are about to destroy and reject this very term—who ask to be able to choose the best, to be able to find quality; for the producers and operators of the world of food, who want to improve and define their professional skills; and for the elderly, who feel uncomfortable in a world that has changed too quickly.

We must provide the tools, convey the information, teach people how to perceive; we must sensitize them and develop values and awareness. We must have at our disposal keys to interpretation, methods, and mental and operative equipment.

The gastronome must no longer be abandoned to his personal struggle against the standardization of food, against unsustainable artifice, against the loss of taste and biodiversity; he must be helped from an early age, directed, encouraged to take possession of his own sensory nature.

The senses and sensitivity; dining and education; experience and information: these are the steps that will help us master reality, enjoy our right to pleasure, and pursue our search for happiness through man's only irreplaceable resource, food.

1.1 From autodidacts to a network of "educated" people

My experience, like that of every modern gastronome since the time of Jean-Anthelme Brillat-Savarin, has been a very personal one, motivated by the desire to experience food and life more fully, to enjoy the company of those who share my enthusiasms, and by the curiosity to know about the histories of food in every part of the world, from my own small town to the remotest corners of the earth. I have had no formal education, except for a few excellent wine-tasting courses (at Beaune, in Burgundy, France). Those lessons among the greatest producers and tasters of the world illuminated me more than anything else; they were the original stimulus that impelled me to desire more, the awakening of my own senses, the experience of the aromas, colors, and tastes of wine—a continual training, based on wine-tasting, comparison, and the study of the characteristics of various grape blends.

Later, it was a short step from the sensorial analysis of wine to that of food: after regaining awareness of your perceptions, you cannot fail to notice the sensory characteristics of any product.

My senses restored me to my taste, they formed that taste. So the desire to know, once I had understood the importance of the raw material and the techniques of production, grew: from the act of tasting, from simple gastronomic criticism, I wanted to get to know the producers, the fields, and the techniques first hand. At that point, it was necessary to come to grips with agronomy, animal husbandry, cooking, the industry, and the traditional crafts. I learned about small differences in technique which translate into differences in taste, differences between varieties and breeds which impose changes on the manner of cooking and on the final result. The knowledge of the raw materials and the production techniques became, to my eyes, essential. The analysis of the final product was no longer enough; one needed a knowledge of its history.

From here, by making this continual search for information, it was easy to realize that the prevailing homogenization of flavors is simply the result of the homogenization of raw materials and techniques owing to the excessive industrialization of the systems of production. I could no longer find certain tastes; I told myself that perhaps I would never be able to experience them again, and so the loss of biodiversity appeared before my eyes with all its most unpleasant and deplorable consequences. The industrial method, the careless production, the lack of concern with taste, and the increasingly polluted soil suggested to me the idea of criteria of sustainability. Then began the search for another kind of information; the field expanded to include the whole world, and I confronted the complexity of this new vision.

It was another short step toward the factors that govern human productivity: if identities and taste are the result of a continual exchange and of profound interactions, surely we should defend not just biodiversity and the products in danger of extinction, but human beings, the communities that produce the food? Why not link them together in a network? Create a *service* which can welcome them, listen to them, enable them to communicate, be ready to help them whenever they need it? Here, then, was another level of education: social research, the study of forms of solidarity and exchange, the study of networks.

The overall picture has been immensely enriched over the years: from the pure sensorial exercise, the spirit of research has led to a struggle against the injustices that afflict the rural world.

But without the initial spark of pleasure and taste, perhaps nothing would have happened, or at least the process would not have been so complete in the end. We would not have reached the final stage, which brought together five thousand farmers, fishermen, nomads, and processors of about a thousand food communities from 130 countries of the world in a single place: the Palazzo di Lavoro in Turin, from October 20–23, 2004. This was the Terra Madre event, to which I will return later (see pp. 201–203), the final stage in a process which must be explained and reconstructed, replicated in various forms, but always starting from sensoriality and going on to embrace all the other spheres of gastronomic knowledge. Only by reawakening our own sensoriality can we understand certain issues. It is a journey in the opposite direction to that which the "militant" environmentalist or the defender of human rights may take. It is a journey that starts from within ourselves and which opens us to the world.

The sharing of these values—which are none other than the interpretation of reality, the assertion of one's cultural dignity and of a system of food production that is better for humankind and for the earth—must eventually lead to a worldwide network of gastronomes. Not one of self-important critics who go from one restaurant to another dispensing judgments and points, but of new gastronomes who produce, eat, associate, and help each other.

And all this cannot be achieved without lifelong education: in taste and in food, in agriculture and in the environment, in tradition and innovation in the food sector. An education in *gastronomic knowledge*. But how is this education to be imparted?

1.2 *Changing the model, starting with schools*
If the gastronome is self-taught, it means that no official educational institution has ever been able to help him much. Indeed, the schools in particular have serious deficiencies from the point of view of nutritional education. Gastronomy does not exist as a subject of study (it must certainly be one of our aims to make it so), and children are only taught superficial notions of nutrition,

which are often counterproductive. The didactic materials used are usually inadequate as well as being boring, repetitive, and abstract, and are seen by children of all ages as a compulsory course that they study with reluctance. Generally, lessons are limited to nutritional tables and videos about what is "good" and "bad" for you (and the products that children like most are always "bad," because they are rich in flavor enhancers: to say that they are bad for you, to ban them, teaches children nothing, and only makes them reject these forms of teaching). There are sermonlike lessons consisting of purely technical advice, which often comes down to notions about how our organism functions and to elementary rules of hygiene.

The pleasure principle is deliberately ignored—not even considered. While rules of nutrition are no doubt correct and need to be explained, they are not enough on their own. In a world where flavor is lost owing to standardization and the disappearance of some kinds of food, where our direct relationship to food grows ever weaker, impeded by countless artificial intermediaries, we must give taste the central position it once had and teach it in a practical way in all schools.

Telling children where the raw material comes from, letting them touch it, handle it, cook it, and eat it themselves, is the most effective method of teaching them about food and taste. Guiding their sensoriality and teaching them to recognize it, so that they can appreciate the products of their own area and the recipes of their own tradition, is the way to teach them about the nutritional culture to which they belong and to equip them with the tools they will need to choose, discriminate, buy, and evaluate different kinds of food.

This educational model, based on tasting and on a direct relationship with the material, must not be the only one; it must not replace the nutritionist and health-oriented approaches. But it is the missing link that is needed to train children's perception of the world about them from an early age. The method of sensorial literacy has already been codified,[48] and it is a revolutionary approach, with an effectiveness that far exceeds even the most sanguine expectations.

Concerning education in food and taste at school, the experience of Slow Food, which has been confirmed in Italy, Germany, the United States, and Japan, is that children are very receptive to teaching methods that involve the pleasure principle. Their capacity for surprise and their still unclouded senses make them open-minded, and they are happy, for example, to be able to taste different cheeses and learn about the production process and the differences between a product made from unpasteurized milk and another made from pasteurized milk.

But this is not the only direct, joyous, and practical method available to children now; the experience of Slow Food (in Australia, the United States, and Italy) has also given rise to the idea of the *school garden*, a vegetable patch in the school, where children learn to grow their own food, to interpret the signs of the changing seasons, and to gather the fruits of the earth so that they can taste, cook, judge, and compare them with those of the supermarket. Sensoriality here broadens out; it embraces work and the relationship with the earth and with the ecosystem. Children can acquire the natural knowledge that is possessed by people who live in close contact with food production (in the country); they can transcend the limits that ensue from the loss of their local dietary model, from the diffusion of the products of agroindustry, from the diminishing practice of home cooking, and from the spread of fast-food establishments (which persistently court them with enticing advertisements and gadgets of every kind).

There is a desperate need for education about sensoriality and about "the land"; our educational aims from the earliest age should be to provide the necessary tools for children to interpret reality, to orient themselves. The failure of schools to teach children about pleasure, gastronomy, food processing, the basics of agriculture, and the nutritional culture that is part of their identity is nothing short of scandalous.

1.3 Continuing education, always

While it is true that cultural ignorance about gastronomy and food begins at school, it is equally true that education must be constant, must last all through life and not be limited to the rudiments that we pick up in our childhood. The separation that has developed between the worlds of food production and food consumption has meant that the last two or three generations have seen the definitive severing of the umbilical cord which provided a link with the earth and its products for anyone who was lucky enough to see with his own eyes the various stages in the production of food: the growing of crops, the raising of livestock, and the later processing. Two generations have grown up in the shadow of industrial products and are no longer able to discriminate among foodstuffs; they do not know how food is produced, and in many cases they cannot even match a raw material with its finished product.

So we must certainly begin with the schools, but above all with the teachers. Many of them are not equipped to teach these subjects; many already belong to the first generation to lack all gastronomic knowledge. The new educational methods must therefore be taught to teachers, too. And it must be taught to parents, both young and not so young, the first children of that food-and-drink industrial revolution which has left us devoid of taste. I do not wish to blame anyone, teachers or parents, but the cultural-gastronomic annihilation which has spread through our society during the last fifty years has by now affected almost all of them.

The wakeup call is for everyone; gastronomic knowledge must be recovered, and we must create the conditions in which it can be passed on. So the schools must also promote educational schemes: evening courses, tastings held by producers—playful and enjoyable events which teach a new, different, complete, and complex kind of knowledge.

It was to meet this need that Slow Food created its Taste Workshops and Master of Food courses. The former are lessons in tasting, held by the producers themselves or by experts in sensorial analysis and in production. Excellent products are chosen, comparisons are made between them, and various aspects of gastronomic diversity are discussed. The separation of the tasting from any nutritional connotation (nobody goes to the Taste Workshops to "eat") makes possible a learning experience that stimulates sensoriality, and that is guided by people who know very well the characteristics of the products being presented in the workshop. The lessons include gustatory analysis, descriptions of the methods of production, and accounts of the region concerned or of the life and skills of the producer. The aim is to create a friendly and convivial discussion, free of technical jargon, but precise in its multidisciplinary gastronomic analysis. In essence, it is an experience of guided pleasure, and it is very rich in knowledge.

The Master of Food courses are designed as a series of workshops and theoretical lectures on different categories of food (bread, pasta, meat, cheese, oil, et cetera): they are a kind of people's university, spread all over Italy (the courses are organized by Slow Food's regional associations). They aim to provide the basis of a comparative knowledge of the taste and production methods of most of our foods. There are twenty "subjects" in all, and everyone who completes the course receives a certificate.

Both of these course programs, unlike conventional wine-tastings or cooking courses, mainly concentrate on sensorial analysis as a means of understanding, as a basis for evaluating productive, territorial, and technical differences. The sensorial analysis, along with the analysis of the production processes, gives a new perspective to the people who participate in these courses; it changes their approach to food and lays the foundations for a new, more conscious way of eating. The search for pleasure is again central and reflected in the style of the lessons: they are informal but precise in their exposition and serious in their approach to tasting; they are playful but rich in ideas, stories, techniques, and cultural stimuli. The teaching is done in a clear, comprehensible language that stimulates people's curiosity about food, sensitizes them to gastronomic and environmental themes, and enables them to meet and talk to producers.

In citing these examples, I do not mean to say that it should be compulsory for everyone to attend Taste Workshops and

Master of Food courses; the important issue is that educational opportunities be provided for all ages and at various times of the day, and that they be *enjoyable*. These courses should embody a new way of discussing food, a new gastronomic language, closer to the sensibility of ordinary people, and more explicit about the everyday facts of our continuous relationship with food. Meetings with producers, for example, are important; they make it possible to draw directly on a source of gastronomic knowledge that is often denied to us, merely because we are often unwilling or unable to access it.

The use of clear language, without too much gourmet's rhetoric or technical jargon, is the first step toward rejuvenating gastronomic science and making it a lifelong educational corpus, which will be made explicit every time we eat. Playful language will create the impression of a different and more light-hearted approach: even giving a workshop a lively title is an indication that the class will not be boring. The participants taste foods, compare them, learn about production techniques, and get to know the producers in an informal atmosphere, and the lesson is conducted in everyday language, in a manner that is simple and playful, without being foolish or trivial.

1.4 Flying high, with no sense of inferiority

Sensorial analysis, learning about production methods, and comparative tastings are the basis of that education in gastronomy, food, and taste that is lacking in schools and in society as a whole. A strategy of change for the food system starts with the creation of courses in public and private schools at all levels, for all ages, which will form the basis for reacquiring sensorial lucidity, criteria of judgment, and the elements of gastronomic culture.

But beyond this basic level, there are two other educational levels which have to be reached in order to restore full centrality to food in our society and make it a tool, everywhere, of cultural and economic growth and of an improvement in the quality of life. We have seen that quality is made up of three aspects: good, clean, and fair. Besides culinary pleasure and its conscious practice, there are many other aspects which are related to the production of our food; these include methods of production and sustainability, whether ecological, economic, or social. Obviously, the input of the courses that teach people to taste, to recognize, and to interpret the techniques of production will not be enough on its own. In order to make choices of quality, the consumer must have at his disposal all the information he needs to be able to recognize quality, and he does not always find assistance in this search. Labeling systems are often inadequate or cryptic; the traceability of the production process of a product is often interrupted or conceals dark corners, doubtful provenances, and strange commercial operations. In many cases, it is impossible to get back to the precise raw material. The environmental costs of production are unknown, and we have no way of knowing if social injustices are being perpetrated (if this does happen, it will certainly not be mentioned on the label).

The educational process runs the risk of, on the one hand, coming up against the impossibility of knowing factors which are crucial for judgment and choice, and on the other, restricting itself to the evaluation of a few products and not examining everyday practice. There must be a continual stimulus to curiosity and to an interest in all the "gastronomic" aspects of quality. There must be a desire to know more and more, the "political" will to bring pressure to bear to ensure that information is provided and that the processes of production are made as transparent as possible.

A second educational level is thus left to the actions that the consumer can make in his everyday relationship with shopping and meals, and it depends on a greater flow of information about all that is food. This information must be requested, demanded, and then used.

The third level is the highest one, which has legitimate claims to a cultural dignity recognized at the academic level and forms an integral part of the world of knowledge. If it is accepted that gastronomy is a science, not the private concern of autodidacts but a multidisciplinary scientific body of knowledge that requires a familiarity with a variety of disparate disciplines, then that science should be fully recognized as such and studied and taught in universities.

The first college of gastronomic sciences has already been founded: the University of Gastronomic Sciences of Pollenzo and Colorno,[49] which was strongly supported by Slow Food (I apologize for the continual references in this chapter to the association of which I am president, but our overall educational project is designed according to the various instructional needs that I am presenting here, and I cannot find many other examples that can give an idea of this philosophy and of the strategies that need to be applied). This institution is the first experiment in the world that has set out to provide at university-level courses which use the senses, the experience of culinary phenomena, and the concretization of products as the basis for speculation about food.[50] It embraces and links both humanistic and technical-scientific subjects, freeing every discipline from the traditional study methods to create an approach that is open to all matters concerning food and which takes its point of departure from *experience*. Experience—travel, training courses, visits, tastings, exercises, interviews with operators—is equivalent, in the new university, to what preparatory courses are in traditional education. Experience is the foundation on which all theoretical knowledge is built; it will provide the basis for readings and advanced study, and for incursions into other fields of knowledge. This is the first organic attempt at teaching taste, which is suspended in that limbo between objectivity and relativism, where the private mingles with the public and flavor with knowledge. The gastronome's task is to move along these borders, to learn how to do so; that is what a university of gastronomic sciences must teach.

If, as one hopes, other university courses are founded elsewhere, the field will be widened and the number of schools of thought in gastronomic science will increase, and we will begin to see the emergence of new teachers, new scholars, and new forms of awareness. If gastronomy succeeds in attaining the academic esteem that it deserves, we will be able to introduce it into the schools as well, and into all the stages of an education which must continue throughout a person's life. People will finally cease to consider only the sole definition of "food science" that has been regarded as valid until today, with its dual sense of the physiology of nutrition and industrial production: the cold, detached study of food, of its industrial standards, composition, and nutritional value.

Gastronomic science is very different: it involves the study of taste, provenance, value, and quality; it does not keep the relevant disciplines apart, but encourages the exchange and circulation of knowledge. It consciously abandons the traditional characteristics of an academic education, while asserting its legitimate right to academic status.

1.5 *Educating and being educated*

Rejuvenating and simplifying the technical language, accepting multidisciplinary complexity, basing research on the senses and experience, and getting to know the producers, their techniques, and the characteristics of the areas and ecosystems: these are the main aims of a new educational methodology which is needed in order to create new gastronomes and carry out the collective daily search for quality. It is a lifelong education—one to be savored, one that teaches pleasure and makes pleasure its watchword, one that is easy to transmit and to communicate. We are only at the beginning of this process, but I believe that by continuing to stress the importance of education and by carefully planning its structures and methodologies, we will be able to bring about a new connection between earth, food, and man. This new relationship can be fully shared by everyone—as if there were a gastronome in all of us, leading us to no longer just be *consumers*, but something different, more interesting, more intelligent, and happier.

Between 1996 and 1998, Slow Food developed the the Ark of Taste: an idea for cataloguing all the products threatened with extinction and promoting them, so that as many people as possible would strive to save them. After its applauded launch in the Salone del Gusto of October 1998, the Ark had great success, not only in Italy but also abroad; indeed, even today its international commission works untiringly to identify products that need to be put on the list.

However, after the Salone del Gusto of 1998, we were forced to reflect on how concretely to save this endangered heritage, and it was then that the idea of Presidia was born. These are small-scale projects devoted to the preservation of specific food products, carefully selected and diversified according to the kind of intervention that is required (to give some examples: financing for producers, the building of infrastructures, marketing, and the activation of commercial networks). But in order for the idea to be practicable, some prototypes had to be designed, and the first was that of the capons of Morozzo.

It happened very quickly: I always like to visit the traditional agricultural fairs of my region. In addition to attending the Fiera del Bue Grasso (Fair of the Fat Ox) at Carrú, which is every year on the second Thursday in December and has become an institution, for several years I had also been going to a smaller event, which is held annually in the same pre-Christmas period in the little village of Morozzo. Here, the women raise magnificent capons with superior sensory characteristics.

By 1998, however, the fair had become a depressing occasion. Since the rural economy had completely changed in that area, the tradition of the capon had been dying out. Few women raised them anymore, and the buyers were even fewer—and that, despite the time of year, which should have been one of feasting. In fact, the onerous practice—it took great expertise and passion—of raising these birds was no longer repaid by a just price, and the fair had degenerated to a very sad echo of times past.

After that experience, I became convinced that the only way to keep the tradition of the capons of Morozzo alive was to carry out a commercial operation that guaranteed the women a fair price. I decided to propose to them that they raise a thousand capons for the following year, which I would undertake to buy at a price almost double that paid in 1998 (24,000 lire a kilo instead of 13,000 lire).

So it was that in January 1999, I invited all the poultry farmers to the hall of the village council of Morozzo to make my offer. The women sat there with folded arms while their husbands stood around them, forming a frame; I took the floor and made my proposal. I told them that they must not give up and that I would give them my personal assistance, by trying to involve as many friends as possible in what would be a sort of sale *en primeur*, as is customary with wine. The atmosphere was somewhat tense; I still remember those rustic faces, used to hardship, which had little confidence in me and barely a glimmer of hope. Their incredulity was understandable: the townie's offer must have sounded rather strange. They probably thought that I was either trying to swindle them or was a mad philanthropist.

Indeed, it did prove difficult to carry out the operation, and if I kept my word it was due not only to my stubborn determination but also to a network of friends who agreed to spread the news and do the selling. It was not easy: for example, my friend Enzo Ercolino, a great producer of wine from southern Italy with a wonderful sense of humor, came all the way up to Piedmont to buy two. His wife, Mirella, added up the bill and, what with the journey and such a high price, she asked him, in amiable reproof, what kind of bargain he thought he had made. The bargain was that he had helped to save the capons of Morozzo from extinction, because it was on that occasion that the spell was broken and people began to understand that the added value of these quality products deserved to be recognized.

The group of people who participated in the enterprise (try to imagine selling a thousand capons at twice the market price!) had become the protagonists of the scheme as much as the producers. They had become co-producers, and word of mouth plus personal commitment was enough to save the capons for good. Today, the fair is prosperous and well-attended, and I am sure that the scenes I witnessed in 1998 will not be repeated.

From that moment, Presidium by Presidium, the Slow Food movement began to work with productive know-how, with the agricultural economy, with food marketing, with agroeconomy, animal husbandry, fish farming, and milk and cheese processing—simply drawing on the knowledge of rural people and evaluating the resulting characteristics of their products.

We were not mere consumers—we had taken responsibility for part of the production system, if only from the cultural point of view: we had become co-producers. Every time I see statistics showing the increased profitability of Presidium products that are no longer in danger of extinction, I remember the looks I was given in January 1999 by those inhabitants of Morozzo, where today I know for certain that production has become more sustainable from all points of view and that some young people have undertaken to carry this economy forward in a spirit of respect for food quality.

....

2. CO-PRODUCERS

The complexity of the gastronomic subject matter and the desire—both for reasons of personal gratification and for the health of the planet—to seek good, clean, and fair quality when shopping for food make the life of what is generally termed the "consumer" very hard. The quantity of information that has to be obtained and the educational effort (of the senses, the sensibility, and the intellect) that has to be made can have the effect of confusing people, of tiring them so much that they just give in and become passive toward methods of production that are unsustainable for taste, for the environment, and for society. Consuming today is difficult, perhaps even more difficult than producing. But one must not give in; one must reconsider and redefine the role of the consumer, starting with the term itself.

The *consumer* originates with the consumer society: the consumer consumes. But he does not consume only the goods that he buys; he consumes earth, air, and water. This *consumption*, if maintained at its present rate, will lead to destruction of resources. The very act of production involves consumption: often, calculating all the kinds of possible cost (including those external to the mere production process), one cannot fail to notice that the balance sheet is in the red. It is not my intention to denounce the capitalist system in itself, nor to inveigh against "filthy lucre," but this word "consumer" unfortunately conceals mistaken models, a mistaken approach, which can only be rectified with the greatest effort. The word itself shows this: "consuming," which has become part of everyday language, no longer manages to conceal its true meaning—that of wearing out, using up, destroying, progressively exhausting.

So we must change our attitudes, starting with our terminology. *Consuming* is the final act of the production process; it should be seen as such, and not as extraneous to the process. The old consumer must therefore begin to feel in some way part of the production process—getting to know it, influencing it with his preferences, supporting it if it is in difficulty, rejecting it if it is wrong or unsustainable. The old consumer, now the *new gastronome*, must begin to feel like a *co-producer*.

It will be the producer's responsibility to accept him as such, so as to create a new community of aims, a new *productive community* with food at its center (which we will call *food com-*

munities), and a single and fundamental value, the desirable sum of the values necessary for it to be produced and co-produced in a way that is good, clean, and fair.

2.1 Cutting the umbilical cord

The immense distance, the absolute separation between the producer and the consumer, between the phase of production and that of food consumption, is a fairly recent phenomenon and is growing. The production methods of food of the industrial kind—and most of all, the quantitative, reductionist, and utilitarian philosophies that they imply—are the main causes, both direct and indirect.

The effect of these styles has been that knowledge about production has become specialized and technologized to the point where it is incomprehensible to anyone who is not directly responsible for it. They have hidden the places of production away in large factories and centralized them, removing them from view and erasing them from the common reality that is experienced by most people. They have processed the natural material to the point where its original characteristics are unrecognizable. They have brought about the commoditization of every phase, from cultivation to distribution, monopolizing all knowledge (agricultural, processing, and commercial) and presenting the consumer with a finished, packaged product, processed by incomprehensible and unexplained techniques, and bought like any other consumer article, under a brand name. The brand name stands as a surrogate for the real characteristics of a product; it becomes a surrogate for knowledge. They have left us, after a mere fifty years, confused, frightened (thanks to phenomena like mad cow disease), and unable, except through a slow and laborious process of learning, to understand and judge food for ourselves.

But food, as we have seen, is far more than a simple product to be *consumed*: it is happiness, identity, culture, pleasure, conviviality, nutrition, local economy, survival. To think of stripping it of all these values, of all the connotations that a mouthful of food can immediately convey, to think of mediating and reducing these connotations to the point where they disappear, is one of the greatest follies ever conceived by man.

Before the onset of this revolution, which has left us ignorant and unable to taste, the situation was quite different. The basic knowledge about food, its provenance, its processing and cooking, used to be handed down from generation to generation in an almost physiological manner. The country life, but also the proximity of town dwellers to the raw materials, through the relationship they established with the producers at the market or with the local shopkeeper, fostered a natural learning process. Family practice would teach without formal lessons; children saw their fathers cut up the animals for meat and collect the products from the vegetable garden, and watched their mothers make preserves and cook every day, according to the season. How many people today know the names of the various cuts of meat by heart? How many know how to make a good preserve?

There was a sort of umbilical cord that was guaranteed by the proximity between agricultural practice, processing, and consumption. Many activities of this productive cycle were the appanage of the consumer himself, who was thus in effect a *co-producer*. This was not just a prerogative of the rural world; in the town, the same thing happened—whether it was a legacy of recent life in the country, contact and the exchange of knowledge and information between the producer and the townsman was manifested in the shops and markets.

Nowadays, that umbilical cord has been cut, and dramatically so. Opening a packet of pasta in sauce, which we only need to heat up for a few minutes in a saucepan, makes us forget, neglect to think about what kind of pasta we are eating, what tomatoes were used in the sauce, what other ingredients went into that dish and what their history has been.

Consuming no longer has anything to do with producing, because the system of food distribution, which is riddled with paradoxes, has interposed itself, ever more intrusive, titanic, and centralized.

In this case, too, innovations have given the impulse: increasingly powerful, rapid, and refined methods of preservation; the cold chain of refrigerated delivery systems, means of transport and logistics. If Nicolas Appert or Francesco Cirio may legitimately be numbered among the benefactors of mankind, with their inventions in canning and sterilization methods, the principle that inspired them has been transformed with increasing speed until it has become paradoxical: consuming a poor-quality fish caught in the Indian Ocean today is easy, accessible, but unsustainable. Milk remains "fresh" for weeks thanks to highly sophisticated techniques, and the law now allows even long-life milk to be called "fresh"; you don't know where it comes from, and it generates inefficient and pollutant distribution systems. (Where is the sense in hundreds of trailer trucks carrying milk all over Italy from a single factory, which has already collected that milk from all over the country after an equivalent number of previous journeys? Would it not be more logical and cleaner to make milk travel the shortest possible journey, so that it is always fresh and locally produced?)

If industry has deprived us of knowledge, the distribution system has accentuated this expropriation, to the point where it has made the provenance of products impossible to trace. The word traceability, which is a must for every self-respecting food production chain nowadays, hardly existed ten years ago. Before mad cow disease and the dioxin-contaminated chicken, it was not possible to trace the place of production of the raw material for industrial products. It is still very difficult to discover in which field a lettuce served in a fast-food restaurant was picked, even though the lettuce is described as being of "national" origin: national, yes, but where did it come from exactly? From what kind of cultivation? What preservatives was it treated with? What was the cost of the transport, and of any human activity involved? It must be admitted that there has now been a slight reversal in the trend, at least as far as the statements of intent of many large-scale producers and distributors are concerned, but the distance between the agricultural origin and the place of consumption is now so great that it will take a considerable effort to guarantee a system of traceability for all products.

This is not to say that we should all go back to living in the country or to producing our food ourselves, but the severed umbilical cord must be repaired—through the search for information, through a commitment by the producers to provide information about their processes and their transportation of raw materials, through a willingness on the part of the large-scale distributors to redesign their system to achieve greater localization, through us and our desire to become co-producers again as we once would have been as a matter of course, and through our efforts to set up new food communities, in which the new gastronome is simply the final link, but an essential one in the whole chain. Food communities should unite producers and co-producers where both parties feel, and operate, as *new gastronomes*.

2.2 Agricultural and gastronomic acts

Wendell Berry, fine poet that he is, has condensed into a single phrase the whole meaning of being a co-producer: "Eating is an agricultural act." We should adopt these words and make them our motto, for they condense the whole awareness that, by our choices as the final consumers in a long process that starts from the land, we influence production, the styles of management of the earth and the environment, as well as the future of farming communities. It also conveys all the solidarity, the sense of *community*, almost of belonging, that we should feel toward the producers of our food. Bringing them closer to us, physically and also psychologically, is a mission for the new gastronome.

But the sense of community must be shared by the producers, with awareness and through the most complete openness. To paraphrase Berry, therefore, one might also argue that "cultivating, stock-raising, and processing must be a gastronomic act." The system of consumption that has become dominant, the distancing of the person who makes from the person who eats, has led to such a mutual separation that there is actually a conflict, an antagonism, between producer and consumer. Alone and disconnected, the producers are in the hands of those who control the intermediate processes. On the one hand, there are situations like the one that occurred recently in Italy, when the retail prices of produce rose steeply while the growers complained that wholesale prices were lower than they had ever been; on the other hand, there are the great global distortions, whereby small farmers produce goods that travel around the world to end up on somebody else's plate after an untraceable process, leaving the farmers in abject poverty.

The producers are at the mercy of this system just as much as the consumers, and many have lost the taste of the land: dispossessed of their knowledge and expertise, they have found themselves abandoned to the agribusiness industry. The latter supplies them with seeds, fertilizers, chemical treatments, animal feed, and antibiotics, which are then simply *applied* to the land and the animals. In many cases, the producers are nothing more than factory workers, with no relationship with the earth.

Farmers used to be connected to the land.[51] But it is not like that any longer. We are faced with people who live on a production line, feeling as alienated as Charlie Chaplin did in *Modern Times*, people who do piecework in the cattle sheds, in the huge fields, giving *medicine* to the earth and the animals, so that production and sales will be as high as possible, whatever the means. No matter if the earth dies, no matter if the food is not genuine and *natural*, no matter if it is tasteless. The farmer in these cases *doesn't know* who will eat it, and the production is completely *industrial*: a scale economy. Someone raises hundreds of Holstein cows packed together in a large shed; he gives them fodder specially designed to make them produce as much as possible and feeds it to them by pressing a button on the automatic control system connected to the storage silos; he milks them in almost continuous rotation with machinery that conveys the milk into cisterns that are picked up by big trucks, and his profits increase with even the tiniest increase in production per cow: this man is like Chaplin's factory worker. He has no respect for the consumer (whom he does not know and does not want to know) or for the quality of the milk. He has no respect for himself and for the role he might have as a producer of food.

Growing accustomed to producing in this manner, within a couple of generations the farm worker loses his own senses, too, and the deterioration in his relationship with nature is likewise translated into what he eats; once, though poor, he was not willing to do without taste—traditional country cooking proves that—whereas today in order to eat he mingles with the consumers among the shelves of the nearest supermarket, filling his cart with awful food that has no taste. The farmer, just like the consumer, is deprived of his senses; he is no longer the master of his life and of his future.

On the one hand, then, we have producers who are alone and confused and who mingle with the consumers, and on the other hand, consumers who are alone and confused. Everyone consumes in the world; those who produce know nothing of gastronomy; those who consume know nothing of agriculture; those who are concerned with ecology do not connect it with food; wealth is unevenly distributed and knowledge disappears.

In this scenario, power lies with the distributors, with the intermediaries, with the people who provide the farmer-cum-factory worker with his materials (seeds and so on), and the people who create the brand name of the final product, which is untraceable and unrecognizable except through advertising. (Significantly, such advertising always tries to simulate a certain naturalness: bottles of olive oil picked from trees, ecological oases in vague, unidentifiable locations, plentiful ears of wheat on the packets of sliced bread). The case of financial holding companies—which simultaneously own animal feed factories, systems of animal-rearing in agistment,[52] trucks, sausage factories, dairies, and major interests in supermarket chains—is the clearest indication of this elusive industry, whose connections are administered by a few individuals.

This system must change, and there is only one figure who can unite and concern everyone: the *new gastronome*. The term is as applicable to farmers who have a gastronomic sensibility as it is to the co-producers (consumers who are aware that "eating is an agricultural act"). Both are on the same level, as leading figures in food production who seek all the dignity they deserve. To achieve this aim, they must educate themselves to be new gastronomes, but must also succeed in transcending distances of every kind and feeling part of a community—a food community but also a "community of destiny," of common destiny.

2.3 Near and far

The distance that has opened up between producers and consumers is not just an abstract distance, represented by the total lack of communication—and often near antagonism—between them, but also by the fact that they live in different worlds, both clouded by the philosophy of profit and unbridled consumerism.

The distance is physical, perceptible, and difficult to transcend.

To feel that one is a co-producer, it is necessary to work on this physical distance, which is a consequence of the processes of globalization (food products can make very long journeys before they end up on our plates), and on the antagonism, the increasingly strong polarization between town and country. For industrial agriculture is basically an urban invention. The consumers in the towns, together with those who have designed the system to oblige them, have in effect determined the kind of agriculture that exists today—and in much of the world, this has been a choice based on ignorance caused by physical and cultural distance from the places of production. Farmers have been forced to accept the system, because they depend on the market. So it may be assumed that if there is room for a new agriculture, this, too, will have to be an urban invention, but one based on an alliance, and on proximity, between the people of the country and the town. This is obviously a question that implies the renewal of local economies and a shortening of the food production chain.

In more practical terms, we must begin to adopt an approach of "local adaptation."[53] This is a principle that has always been practiced by every living species on the planet, and there seems to be no reason why the human species should be exempt from this necessity. In the past, we did so because we had no choice: agriculture was adapted to the territory because there was no other alternative. Then we moved away from this principle because nature gave us cheap fuel and the economic rule became "if you cannot get it here, you can get it somewhere else." But when this method is no longer viable—and we are very close to that point— we will have to think again and adapt locally. This means that we will once again have to consider what potential and what limitations an area has. We will have to consider which productive *communities* exist and how they can provide for our nutrition.

This concept is closely linked to that of subsistence, or the ability of the people of an area to live on their own resources. One of the factors that accelerated the transition to industrial agriculture, as far as farmers are concerned, was that of persuading families to give up the subsistence generated by their small agricultural businesses. Quite the contrary, the rule ought to be that every state or community must first and foremost think of feeding itself, and only when this aim has been achieved should it think about trade. This rule obviously has different implications according to the part of the world that is under consideration. To take the most extreme cases, in the poorest areas, which are predominantly rural, it will be the basis of a dignified life, of guaranteed survival in harmony with tradition and the surrounding environment, and it will be a precondition for possible sustainable development. In the rich areas, which are predominantly urban, the rule can be applied with a (theoretically) simple localization of products, with the search for the closest products (as in the research into the impact of food miles) through the creation of direct buying groups, formed in conjunction with farmers (community-supported agriculture, called CSAs), or with the creation of more farmers' markets.

The idea of urban buying groups at the local level, for example, should be developed and implemented. American and French experiments (there are also a few isolated Italian cases) have shown that they work, and that they are an excellent way of bypassing unfair and unsustainable distribution systems. Groups of city dwellers get together with groups of farmers to meet their respective needs: the city dwellers want fresh, seasonal products at a good (fair) price and want to be able to know the person who grows them; the farmers need to have the guarantee of a fair price, not to be at the mercy of fluctuations in the market, and want the fruits of their production to be appreciated with "gastronomic" sensibility and not confused, diluted, or eliminated by the distribution and market systems. They agree on a price that satisfies both parties: the city dwellers pay in advance for the whole year's produce and in exchange the farmers agree to deliver fruit, vegetables, meat, and cheese to their homes every week. It is the ideal solution for both parties and, as may be noted, all that is needed is a little goodwill and a spirit of sharing or, if you like, co-production.

The problem, essentially, is to relocate production and consumption so that they are in the same places—geographical areas that are not too large. The facilities offered by transport and by the now globalized food system could meet any serious deficiencies, compensate for any imbalances, harmonize the system, and guarantee the services essential to the "producing communities." The same may be said of the new means of communication; from this point of view the Internet is a frontier with immense potential that has yet to be fully explored.

We must revive the system of local adaptation, we must relocate, and we must be aware that food is a *network* of co-production, where knowledge is shared and methods of production are sustainable. Food must be seen as a network, which thus forms another network, consisting of food communities.

2.4 Communities

On the preceding pages, we have introduced the concepts of *producing communities* and *food communities*. It would be best to explain the difference, so that no confusion arises later.

Take a dish of pasta with tomato sauce. Look at it. Try to imagine (unless you are so fortunate as to already *know*) the wheat from which the pasta was made, the tomatoes that make up the sauce, the basil that aromatizes it, the parmesan that makes it more tasty. Imagine the people who sowed and processed the plants, the animals that gave that milk, the people who milked them, the people who reaped the wheat. Think of the places of provenance: traditions, cultures (the wheat was Ukrainian or Canadian; the tomatoes Spanish; the basil Ligurian; the parmesan ... well, at least that was traceable), societies, economies. Think of the history: tomatoes brought to Europe from America; the pasta, whose method of production is the result of an exchange between Arabs, Chinese, and Italians. Imagine the journeys, the transport, the processing, the packaging that those products have been subjected to. Think back to your purchases, where you bought them, how you brought them home, and which hands—yours?—cooked that pasta.

Food is a *network*: of men and women, of knowledge, of methods, of environments, of relations. The multidisciplinary nature of gastronomy makes it possible to interpret it, analyze it, evaluate it, and perhaps even know the other people who make up the network.

In accepting the principle of co-production, the new gastronomes are part of that network, together with the producers, who also have *gastronomic* aims. The people who make up the network should in theory all have the same gastronomic aim: that this dish of pasta, for example, be good, clean, and fair.

The people who make up the network thus have a common aim, and so they are a community—a virtual one if you like, but a community nonetheless. This is what we mean by a *food community*. The idea can be expressed at various economic levels, which include the "producing communities." A producing community may be one that links together individual producers—say, for example, farmers who are dedicated to the growing of a rare variety which they save from extinction by making it economically healthy. A producing community may be a national consortium of small fishermen who fight for the recognition of their right to fish. A food community, on the other hand, might be a community of farmers and city dwellers who form a buying group (CSA, community-supported agriculture) or a group of associated gastronomes who want to exchange knowledge about food.

These communities (food and producing) are more or less closely interlinked right up to the highest, planetary level: the "community of destiny." The producing communities and the food communities (of producers and co-producers) may therefore be local or global: they apply the principle of local adaptation, but they feel that they are sisters to all the other communities that operate in any part of the world. Every new gastronome (both the producer and the co-producer) is aware of sharing a destiny, and aware, too, that this destiny is determined by the choices each person makes, which he hopes will be good, clean, and fair. We are talking, of course, about the destiny of the earth, which the reports of scholars tell us is gravely ill, economically unbalanced, increasingly hurried, and sad.

The food community (which, it should be remembered, may also include the producing community) operates on the land. It is represented through the knowledge of its members and of what they do, but it may cut across strict localization: it may be made up of people who are united by their work and situated in a particular area, but it may also comprise people united by the fact that they constitute a complete production chain, reaching as far as the consumer, or rather co-producer. They are all concerned to ensure that the distances, physical and psychological, become as short as possible, and that at the same time there is no kind of isolation between the different realities: we are all gastronomes.

Even if I do not consume the quinoa of a small producing community of Peruvian farmers, I must feel that I am their co-producer, share their aims, adhere in principle to their project of social redemption and defense of biodiversity. Being a great consumer of the San Marzano tomatoes of Campania, I am a co-producer of the farmers who saved them from extinction at great personal sacrifice. If I buy apples at the market directly from the farmer, I had better meet him, speak to him, and ask how he grows them, because I want to be his co-producer. I belong to various realities, but at the same time to one alone; to various *food communities*, but to a single *community of destiny*.

Vandana Shiva, who became a close friend of mine after the meeting in Florence described in Diary 6, pressed me for at least two years to go to India to visit the projects that her association, Navdanya, runs all over the country. The excuse each time was an invitation to give a lecture as part of an event Navdanya organizes every year in October in New Delhi, in memory of a person whom I had never heard of until a short time ago: Sir Albert Howard. In 2004, I finally accepted the invitation, also taking the opportunity to pay a visit, in advance of Terra Madre (see pp. 201–203), to the Indian communities that would be coming to Turin, and to carry out the official launch of Slow Food in India.

In order to prepare my New Delhi lecture, I decided to learn about Howard by reading his biography and his major work: *An Agricultural Testament.*[54] I was immediately fascinated by this man, who lived and worked in India over half a century ago, having been sent there by the British government in his capacity as a botanist, with the task of studying methods to improve the local agriculture. In fact, he ended up improving British agriculture by transferring from India the traditional organic techniques of the farmers he met. His book is still today a very modern work, notable for the intellectual honesty of its approach in a world where Western agronomic science usually tries to impose its visions and strategies on others.

Learning about the ideas and techniques described by this great British scientist and seeing how he approached the Indian cultures and farming practices, drawing lessons from them, made a strong impact on me. His book, published in 1940, would be worthy reading for present-day farmers all over the world: at the center of all agricultural practice, Howard insists on preserving the fertility of the soil, which must be maintained with noninvasive methods and on no account polluted with chemicals. Equally impressive was Howard's respect for traditional culture; it is a very un-Eurocentric approach from a man who listens with humility and even extols the virtues of work methods that are in some respects considered archaic.

The discovery of this man, and the realization of what he still represents today for the Indians who are fighting for clean agriculture, in harmony with their own traditions and with biodiversity, was a very important experience for me—the demonstration that a "dialogue between realms" (modern science and traditional science) can exist and be fruitful. Howard's attitude contains the basic premise for creating this dialogue: listening. If you know how to listen, you know how to conduct a dialogue. That, above all, is what I have learned from Howard and from my firm friendship with Shiva. It is a great moral lesson, which encourages the meeting and peaceable exchange between different visions.

After all, we know next to nothing about the rest of the world: New Delhi, for example, teems with variegated life, enveloped in incredible perfumes: the city gave me some extraordinary taste experiences and never disappointed me at any stage of that important trip. In the end, I concluded that we Westerners are truly ignorant. From the culinary point of view, I was able to appreciate the skill of the peasant women whose wondrous cooking left me astonished and full of admiration.

I can fully support something that chef Ferran Adrià told me, an experience he had which he takes as a warning against the temptations of grandeur. After he was named the best chef in the world by the *New York Times*, he was taken to China by the Spanish ambassador and introduced to some magnates of the Chinese food-and-drink industry. The Chinese eyed him inscrutably: one of them, unable to restrain himself, scoffed in an undertone, "So this is the best chef in the West!"

The fact that in India I ate at peasant tables, encountering the same expertise and feeling the same pleasure that the great chefs can give, is probably an indication that our very idea of cuisine, graded into high, middle, and low, needs to be revised, indeed overturned. But where are the great Indian chefs, if in the poorest classes the cooking is so good? The Western criteria of judgment, which have degenerated into a system of rankings and points and a rather snobbish kind of gastronomic criticism, would be of no use here, for the simple flavors of the peasant women of the Punjab and the vast pre-Himalayan plain catapulted me into a dimension that I will never be able to describe.

I think this was the underlying element which many years ago captivated the intellectual honesty of Howard, who could do nothing but listen and learn, having realized that he had nothing to teach.

....

3. DIALOGUE BETWEEN REALMS

The situation in which the earth finds itself is very serious. I do not want to sound like a scaremonger, but something is definitely wrong, and we must think again about which way to turn the tiller that steers us toward the future.

Quantitative and reductionist thought are not in themselves the problem. The scientific method, though it denies that some senses are useful to the interpretation of reality,[55] is not in itself the problem. It is the distortions of these modes of thought and their predominance over everything else that have created an unsustainable situation.

The increasing speed of the world, which imposes on us ever-accelerating rhythms of life, work, and thought, accentuates the existing distortions, and the complexity around us threatens to overwhelm us. Since speed has become the dogma of modern life, we are compelled for the sake of our survival not to think too much and to discard anything that seems to slow us down. Moreover, the consumer society merely justifies the creation of new "garbage"; it justifies waste and the discarding of anything that seems unproductive or "slow." Anything that is of no use (people, cultures, countries) is rejected.

The gastronome cannot fail to notice that this impedes his quest for the good, clean, and fair, and he will have no difficulty, with his desire to work for a better quality of life and food, in identifying the elements from which to begin, on which to base a new lifestyle, a new planetary awareness, and the new people with whom to exchange ideas and form fruitful alliances. Does the dogma of speed prevent us from pondering, tasting, comparing, and choosing? Better then to start with a slowing down, with a rhythm more suited to the training of the senses, to the calm perception of reality and tastes. Better to take more time to meet the producers, to do the shopping, to cook. Better also to "waste" time—not in the sense of discarding it, like everything that is of no use to the disciples of speed—but by taking the time to think, to "lose yourself" in thoughts that do not follow utilitarian lines: to cultivate the ecology of the mind, the regeneration of your existence.

The quest for *slowness*, which begins as a simple rebellion against the impoverishment of taste in our lives,[56] makes it possible to rediscover taste. By living slowly, you understand other things, too; by slowing down in comparison to the world, you soon come into contact with what the world regards as its "dumps" of knowledge, which have been deemed slow and therefore marginalized. By exploring the "margins" of slowness, you encounter those pockets of supposedly "minor" culture that are alive in the memories of old people, typical of civilizations that have not yet become frantic—traditions that guide the vital work of good, clean, and fair producers and that are handed down after centuries of empiricism and practical skill.

In coming into contact with this "slow" world, you feel a new (or renewed) relish for life, you sense the potential of different methods and forms of knowledge as counterweights to the direction currently being imparted to the tiller that steers our route toward the future. You reassess the elements of consumer culture, and in rural knowledge you discover surprisingly simple solutions to problems which speed has made complex and apparently insoluble.

It seems wrong that this immense cultural heritage which has been generated by humankind should be discarded simply because, carried away by our enthusiasm for continuous economic development (which means only growth, and never real development), we allow it all to be dissipated. Should it all just disappear with the death of the elderly, of the most primitive societies, of certain rural traditions? What is vanishing is a way of living in the world and producing food that is no longer compatible with the rhythm of industrialized economic globalization— a lifestyle that cannot coexist with a capitalism of the most extreme and selfish individualism. What we are left with is the depreciation and deterioration of all common goods: goods such as the earth and water, peace and happiness.

Lifelong *education* and the gastronome's awareness must therefore be placed in a cultural context that allows them to express themselves, to grow, to spread, to become a real strategy of change in the systems of production and consumption—of food, first and foremost, but not only of that. For everything starts with food (contact with reality and our system of life), but everything ultimately has an influence on our food.

This cultural context must include the precious and illuminating value of slowness, as a premise for an equally important recovery of the *traditional knowledge* of country people, of different scientific methods, and of all those forms of knowledge usually held to be secondary. This traditional knowledge constitutes a heritage that urgently needs to be catalogued and preserved, as it is on the verge of being permanently erased. It must be made alive and present again—not in a manner antagonistic to modern, "official" science, to the new trends developing in the globalized world of the new technologies, or to all those elements whose supremacy is causing its demise (industry, for example)—but in order to establish a *dialogue* between different kinds of knowledge from different *realms*, to amalgamate them and accord them all equal dignity and authority.

In short, my wish is for a food industry that enters into dialogue with the methods of processing and with traditional cooking; a modern agronomic science that enters into dialogue with agroecology and traditional knowledge; and a scientific research that does not go only in the direction of productivism but places itself at the service of the producing communities and of small-scale agriculture, combining their respective skills. There must be no predominant plan, and equal authority: neither of the two realms is called upon to demonstrate the validity of the other. It is sufficient that they communicate and put their knowledge at the service of good, clean, and fair food, and of the happiness of us all.

3.1 Slowness

For almost twenty years, the Slow Food movement has made slowness its watchword, declaring this from the very beginning in its *Manifesto*, and going well beyond the advocacy of a different way of eating: "Speed has become our chain; we are all victims of the same virus, the fast life, which distorts our habits, assails us in our very homes, forces us to eat in the fast-food restaurants." The purpose was, and is increasingly, clear:

> *Homo sapiens* must regain his wisdom and free himself from speed, which can reduce him to an endangered species.[. . .] Against the universal folly of the fast life we must choose the defense of calm material pleasure. Against those, the majority, who confuse efficiency with frenzy, we propose the vaccine of an adequate dose of guaranteed sensual pleasures, to be administered in slow and prolonged enjoyment.[57]

It was unusual in 1986 to discuss the damage caused by the fast life, but since then the reports of the United Nations and the Food and Agriculture Organization have made this damage only too clear, and philosophers, sociologists, and economists are beginning to criticize our rushed way of life severely. Today, more than twenty years after the Slow Food *Manifesto*, everyone is praising slowness; the newspapers write about the slow life, slow cinema, slow books, slow money, slow school, and even slow fitness for people who go to the gym! Slowness today is a value, a need which society is beginning to regard as pressing: its defense is no longer something that needs to be justified.

Franco Cassano, a sociologist at the University of Bari, has aptly expressed the reasons in his book *Modernizzare stanca* (Modernization Is Tiring):

> This defense is neither a conservative reflex nor a literary exercise, but has more solid and concrete reasons. The first is that slowness in our society is an experience that requires deviation, requires us to go off the beaten track of cultural commonplaces. It enables us to conceive of the value of worlds different from our own, to escape from that force of gravity which makes a culture incapable of understanding others. [...] There is, however, a more specific reason which encourages us to rediscover the value of slowness today: some experiences which are crucial to our maturity cannot be speeded up, and are only possible if they occur slowly. Crisis, growth, and meditation occur in slowness, just as only in slowness can we perceive the complexity of a problem.[58]

And if the new gastronomy is a highly complex subject, it too requires slowness.

In urging people to slow down, we are asking them to look around with greater interest, to be receptive to the details and flavors of the world. The contrast should not be between slowness and speed—slow versus fast—but rather between attention and distraction; slowness, in fact, is not so much a question of duration as of an ability to distinguish and evaluate, with the propensity to cultivate pleasure, knowledge, and quality.

In urging people to slow down, we are asking them to respect nature and not to appropriate it for their own private gain against the common good. We are asking them to respect others, favoring passion and understanding over the quantity of utilitarian aims, friendship and the joining of forces over economic competition, the public over the private, the gift over trade.

In urging people to slow down, we are aware that "slow knowledge"—thrown out like the proverbial baby with the bathwater because it is considered to be incompatible, inferior to methods useful to a rapid increase in profits—is the knowledge which can restore balance to the world, which produces the good, which does not pollute, which saves cultures and identities, which makes it possible to continue to have a fruitful exchange between the diversities: the true creative force.

This knowledge—in the field of scientific and agronomic research, in the area of support for those who are poorest, in the field of ecology and gastronomy—which is considered to be old-fashioned and obsolete, is really extremely modern, and understanding this modernity will be easier if we allow ourselves to be guided partly by slowness. *Partly* by slowness, because speed is not useless, but it is only useful if it learns to coexist with other rhythms. In this case, too, we must set up a "dialogue between realms," between different rhythms. To quote Cassano again, "Slowness is not only the *past* of speed, but also its future."

For while it is true that someone who is too slow risks being left too far behind, being considered a fool, it is also true that someone who is slow can clearly see the limit, can live with it, understands it. Perhaps the limit is the cipher of slowness; if you know its meaning, you are safe from the perils of speed.

"Slow knowledge," in a world of food production which is dominated by industrial methods, is considered to be the *past* and is disregarded. But in fact it is also the future of food, in a dialectical and nonantithetical relationship with faster, often unsustainable knowledge. It is woven into a network of other traditional skills that urgently need to be preserved and revalued, before we completely lose the joy of living in a world which is still on a recognizably human scale.

3.2 Slow knowledge in the food system
During a conference on agriculture and development, the agronomist Michele Campanari, president of the Consortium of Wines of the Upper Mincio in the Italian province of Mantua, confessed to one of my colleagues:

Thirty years ago, after I graduated, I began to spend a lot of time in the country with small farmers, to whom I explained the theories I had learned from books at the university. My knowledge, based on scientific research and published in specialist texts, seemed without doubt more powerful than the traditional knowledge of the farmers. It was more powerful because it was written down: their traditional knowledge, which had developed over centuries of experience, was not written down anywhere; it simply existed in the minds, in the culture of the farmers. It was easy to impose a change in their habits, to introduce new techniques. The farmers did not put up much resistance to advice rendered authoritative by scientific studies; they simply compared it with what they already knew and accepted it. As time went by, I realized that as a result of these innovations in production techniques, accepted quite passively in the name of scientific dignity, the old knowledge, an integral part of the farmers' life and culture, had diminished and was on the verge of disappearing after only two generations. It is a pity that it has never been written down and that it is being lost, superseded by a "modernity" which owes more to the market than to culture.

This testimony illustrates how, in the name of technology, over the last thirty years a process of cultural annihilation has taken place, leading, especially in the rich West, to the disappearance of the farmers' traditional knowledge. This traditional knowledge was the precious result of a slow evolution rooted in the territory, of a cultural growth which for centuries had always progressed side by side with the ecosystem, with biodiversity, and with the culture of the area in which it had developed. The introduction of extensive industrial techniques has not only, as we have already seen, stressed the soil, polluted the environment, and led to a general deterioration in the quality of food, but it has also caused a traumatic break with the traditional knowledge of the rural population, changing landscapes, lives, environments, and the vital relationship between man and nature.

This new process of destruction is happening today in those places that are considered backward, such as many areas of Latin

America, Asia, or Africa, where in order to stimulate some kind of development, the modern agricultural techniques that have conquered the Western countryside are being introduced.

It is time to stop the annihilation: not in the name of a return to the past, of a foolish and antiscientific conservatism, but out of respect for these farming cultures, which originated and developed in harmony with the places where they are located.

First, we need conservation, followed by the "dialogue between realms." The agroecological school puts the latest scientific discoveries and ancient traditional knowledge on the same level; it enters a culture discreetly, without imposing itself in any way, but setting up a dialectical relationship between new and old forms of knowledge, between elements external to the ecosystem and the existing biodiversity. It is a much less invasive approach than science created in the laboratory and introduced without respect into a precise biocultural context that has evolved only over time.

It is not a question of rejecting all innovation a priori: it is a question of asking ourselves what impact innovation will have on the existing situation and whether our innovative effort should not be concentrated on improving that situation, rather than replacing it completely. To cite an example, once again, quite apart from the ethical, health, and economic arguments against GMOs, why must we passively accept their introduction when it is not compatible with the traditional systems? And above all, why must almost all scientific research go in that direction without considering alternative paths? Why are plans being made for GMOs to be grown in arid zones, while nothing is being done to reduce the greenhouse effect which is desertifying entire fertile areas of the planet?

Today, of all the research projects financed by vast amounts of capital, mainly from private but partly from public sources, hardly any are concerned with preserving, transcribing, and testing traditional farming methods. And what research project actively involves the farmers, the people who live off the earth and are able to draw their (and our) sustenance from it?

It is time to stop, or at least to slow down, and accord traditional farmers and their knowledge the dignity they deserve, by listening to them, recording them, and preserving (where it still exists) their valuable function as a harmonious and direct link with the earth.

Let us look at what we have lost, discarded, and let us not continue this reckless cultural annihilation. Right under our noses there is a treasure: the key that will enable us to start again, *slowly*, with the construction of an agricultural world that meets our real needs. We do not need the accumulation of wealth, but its redistribution; we do not need an increasingly standardized and industrialized global food system, but one based on the diversity of cultures and places, and on the quality that these can express. The treasure is an ancient key, but a surprisingly modern response: it enables us to build a new rurality, and in particular a widespread gastronomic sensibility, which will become an everyday productive exercise and not a mere divertissement for a few fortunate individuals.

That treasure is the "slow knowledge" that lives in the hands and hearts of millions of farmers who cling to their own land, in the hands of cooks who are close to the world of agricultural production, in the traditions of peoples who need to improve their condition by taking their own state as a starting point, not by denying it completely and discarding it.

With slow knowledge, we must conduct a "dialogue between realms," which is not archaistic nostalgia, immobilism, or a rejection of science, but a precise desire to draw on different sources of wisdom. In this regard, Enzo Bianchi, the prior of the monastic community of Bose and a distinguished theologian, as well as a gastronome and the product of a farming culture, has said:

> If we refer to that world [the traditional agricultural world which belongs to the past in the West and to the present in the developing countries] and we do so in a critical manner, with discernment, we can garner the fruits of centuries of experience, many of which have undoubtedly been neglected and discarded. Now we are at the beginning of a new world, which some call the "retreating world." We can no longer stop

and foresee, I do not say the future, but even the day after tomorrow. So it is important to have points of reference in the past, without adopting an archaeological approach, but asking ourselves whether those things, which were part of a certain type of wisdom, can still teach us something about this world that is retreating before us.[59]

3.3 The need to catalogue

It is not a question of stating the prevalence of one kind of knowledge—empirical, qualitative, linked with stimuli like pleasure or simple common sense, and built on a fertile coexistence with the natural world—over the other—quantitative, scientific, strictly mathematical, discarding anything that is incalculable. It is a question of linking these kinds of knowledge in a *network*, of making them mutually useful, or simultaneously useful. Neither should be rejected a priori; our goal is to free ourselves from prejudices, while carefully pursuing quality as I have described it. Now, to carry out this kind of operation, we must undoubtedly begin by taking remedial measures, dipping into the trashcan of discarded knowledge and trying to recover those things that are being marginalized. Such knowledge would be difficult to record in writing, because it would inevitably require outside help from someone who could turn it into a publishable work. But the new video, audio, and computing technologies make it easy to record and preserve this knowledge through interviews with the people who are still involved in the activities. We must start systematically recording traditional knowledge—both establishing links among the people already working in this field and creating new research centers.

This is another indispensable element for implementing a real change in the direction of quality: cataloguing this knowledge, a vital task if we are to be able to study it, develop it, or even just hand it on. The importance of this phase should not be underestimated, and it is absolutely essential that the various forces involved be connected in a network.

In bringing together various producing communities from around the world for professional reasons (such as the Terra Madre event and the Presidium schemes), we soon realized that these men and women possess, by virtue of the fact of living in symbiosis with their home environments, ingenious solutions to highly topical problems. The cultivation of amaranth in the arid areas of Mexico, for example, gets around the problem of drought and generates income and highly nutritious food for subsistence. The preparation and consumption of insects provides protein where it is in short supply and creates an alternative to expensive stock farming, as well as ridding the crops of harmful parasites. Although part of the coastline struck by the 2004 tsunami was a natural paradise that had been exploited for tourist purposes, the local population had traditionally avoided settling there, as if aware of the danger and loathe to live in an area that was not advantageous from the production point of view. The severity on the question of diet of many religious precepts, which at first sight seem dictated by mere superstition, in fact conceal considerations of utilitarianism and self-control in people's relationship with the surrounding environment. Traditional rural knowledge, though not as certain and demonstrable as official science, contains an element of *common sense* which cannot be traced by calculation, which pursues not profit but survival, and in the most effective way possible.

Planning the construction of a sort of "universal encyclopedia" of the expertise accumulated by traditional, agricultural, and consumer cultures is the first step toward a definitive redemption of these kinds of knowledge; it is a modern effort to find solutions within the traditions that have developed over the centuries in individual contexts, as well as by comparing the various traditions with each other. This operation, together with a lifelong education and with the awareness of being part of many communities, but ultimately of one alone, will free us from the yoke that we have imposed on ourselves, that of speed at all costs, and will also help us to rediscover lost oases of happiness. Moreover, it is the greatest form of respect that we can show to others, to those who are different from us, and it avoids any kind of fundamentalism, or what happens whenever "one culture sees the diversity of others as a sickness and itself as the cure."[60]

3.4 A holistic approach

When I speak of the need to catalogue (I will go into more detail about this in the next chapter), recover, and analyze "slow," traditional kinds of knowledge, I do so of course as a gastronome, and I refer in the first instance to gastronomic knowledge: agriculture, cooking, processing, preservation, and sustainable activities. I include the whole range of disciplines which form part of gastronomy, calling for a different epistemological approach from that which is currently most usual.

But I will go further: a recent meeting in Washington D.C. with the directors of the Smithsonian Institution reinforced my conviction that it is absolutely necessary to start considering the agricultural world, and in general the world of food production, within an even more complex picture than that to which we are accustomed. The food system is always part of a wider cultural system, whose manifestations are endangered just as much as biodiversity and traditional farming methods are.

If, from the agroecological point of view, these questions have already been examined in some detail and are supported by a substantial literature, they have not received much attention from the gastronomic, let alone from the cultural, point of view. In fact, the three aspects should be closely interlinked in what I would call a holistic vision (see pp. 221–222), making possible conservation activities that take in the whole environment. Let me make myself clearer: we cannot expect to save a gastronomic heritage without asking ourselves what culture it belongs to, what its most characteristic customs are. The study of local cultures requires this effort too, and indeed an overall understanding of a culture is the first and crucial step toward helping it to recover and survive.

What, for the gastronome, is the central concern of food and agriculture must be supported by a broader vision, and we should therefore include the study and cataloguing of what is generally termed folklore: dance, song, music, dialects, oral traditions, traditional architecture, tools, and other modes of expression, such as ways of accompanying work in the fields. It is right that these manifestations of identity should be studied, or at least kept alive, for they are an integral part of complex systems of agriculture and food production at the local level. To say this and to think on the global level—for example, at the level of the communities of Terra Madre—opens up wider perspectives and implies a commitment different from that which we have undertaken so far. An interest in folksongs, music, and dance is an act of respect toward the communities that produce food. Setting up initiatives that will make it possible for these traditions to remain a living symbol of distinct productive identities is an essential task for anyone who wishes to help the people concerned.

4. BACKWARD IN WHAT SENSE?

To recapitulate, the basis of a strategy that leads back to quality must be the recovery of another dimension, the adoption of slowness as a value external to the prevailing system, as a creative space and a meeting point of those values that are excluded from the system. Slowness is compatible with the exercise of the senses, with *lifelong education*; it restores a sense of communitarian belonging and reinforces it through meetings, assistance, exchange, and gifts. But it also provides a basis for reversing the direction of our thought, which is currently focused almost exclusively on profit and on a frenetic efficiency, alienating us from each other even though we are closer together than ever. A reversal of thought, toward attention rather than unconcern, opens up new scenarios for the gastronome, because it reveals that in diversity lies the force which enables us—or used to enable us—to live with dignity on the earth. The world of "slow knowledge," which can be easily wiped out or consigned to a folkloristic limbo, appears to us with all its renewed potential and demands that we respect, conserve, and use it—not in order to create new hierarchies, but to enable all kinds of human progress to coexist, to go onward with courage and with the determination to keep looking backward, before we lose all orientation and set in motion irreversible processes that will impoverish our resources. The producers of good, clean, and fair food (most of whom are small farmers), those who have not yet been irremediably changed by the severing of the umbilical cord to the earth, possess a knowledge which cannot be learned in school and cannot be calculated with mathematic formulas, but which is the result of a symbiotic relationship with creation that many of us have lost. Many of them therefore, simply as living beings, are a vital resource; it is they who have much to teach us. Listening to them, and supporting their communities, rather than trying to teach them how to live, is a vital task for anyone who cares about the future of food and of the earth.

CHAPTER V

CREATING

Gastronomy is a complex science and, if we study it with a multidisciplinary approach, it enables us to regain our sensoriality and provides us with tools for interpretation, values according to which to work, new traveling companions, and an understanding of reality. It helps us to identify the cultural and productive mechanisms that serve the cause of a fairer and happier world; it prompts us to intervene, in the awareness that we have the ability and opportunity to do so. It makes us creative.

It creates a common sensibility, which leads us all to be active participants (as gastronomes, producers, and co-producers) in the quest for an idea of quality (quality of life and quality in products). This is appropriate not only for our own personal well-being, but also for that of others and of the land. This common sensibility induces us to redefine our behavior and our daily objectives, and it gives a new meaning to gastronomy—or rather, to that which stands at the center of human activities: food itself.

The tools of this research and of this redefinition we have already seen: a complex and redefined science; the notion of good, clean, and fair; the desire to educate ourselves and not to succumb to ignorance of the senses and the intellect; the awareness of belonging to a community of destiny; and the desire to develop a new way of promoting and practicing knowledge. There is a new quest for taste, which includes all these ideas, and which, if it is not to be merely idealistic and impracticable, requires planning and pragmatism.

There is a network from which we can start and which can be made as functional as possible—a network of feelings, aspirations, forces, knowledge, and people.

If we restore food to its rightful place at the center of our lives, we see that food *is* the network, and that it must be strong, transparent, good, clean, and fair. If we are what we eat, we are the network: a pragmatic network, which strives to communicate as much as possible. So we need planning and the desire to act, to realize ideas.

....

After Terra Madre, many of the participating communities invited the staff of Slow Food to visit them. I myself, when I am on my travels, always drop in to see them if I happen to be in the neighborhood, and the first opportunity arose very soon (in November 2004, a month after the event), during a trip to Sweden, where I had gone to meet the local representatives of our movement.

On that occasion, I visited the community of the Sami (usually incorrectly termed Laplanders; few people know that this is an insult: "lapp" means "patch" and is pejorative)—a population of only seventy thousand people who live in a region that has no official borders, Sápmi (most people wrongly call it Lapland), in the north of the Scandinavian peninsula, between Sweden, Norway, Finland, and Russia. The Sami I met are those who attended Terra Madre: a nomadic community (like all Sami) of about three thousand people who follow the herds of reindeer on their migrations. Reindeer are their main occupation, and from them they make many products, such as *suovas*—reindeer meat smoked using a traditional method. *Suovas* is threatened with extinction, and Slow Food is endeavoring to protect it.

We went to visit them in one of their camps of traditional huts (made of planks of wood arranged in a conical shape, with a floor of moss and pine branches—very cozy), near Östersund, one of the southernmost places in Sápmi, where the reindeer come before the winter and are slaughtered.

I listened to the long and troubled story of the Sami, while sitting by the fireside in one of their huts. (Many of today's Sami have modernized; they live in prefabricated cottages which they can move, and they follow the reindeer on motor-powered sledges; it would be absurd not to accept these modern advances in a place where the winter lasts for two hundred days a year and where the temperature falls as low as thirty degrees below zero Celsius.) I was also lucky enough to taste some delicious bread toasted over the fire with *suovas*, an excellent product with great commercial potential.

My guide during my visit was the president of the Sami Parliament, a multinational body that represents them in their relations with all other institutions, and I must say that I was delighted with their joy and interest at having participated in Terra Madre. I spent nearly two whole days with them, and we traveled across the very inhospitable but almost magically fascinating area around which the Sami move all year, following the reindeer. It seems almost impossible that in countries like the Scandinavian ones, there can still exist a nomadic population that makes nomadism its raison d'être and is fiercely proud of it. I heard them talk of the injustices they suffer in each state they travel through, of their struggles for right of way in certain areas (when in fact the movement of their herds has an ecological function, though they are not welcomed by the local farmers), of their extraordinarily rich and interesting cosmology, which illustrates how important this kind of knowledge mingled with myth can be. For example, the Sami knew long before Galileo that the earth goes around the sun: it is one of the fundamental concepts of their religion!

On the last afternoon, when the sun had already fallen below the horizon (this happens at about three o'clock in November) and we were strolling along in total darkness, I asked the president of the Sami how they had liked Terra Madre. With evident enthusiasm he said something very illuminating: he told me that no one had ever done so much for the nomadic peoples, and that they were laying the foundations for a kind of international association of such peoples, so that they could all keep in contact and help each other to cope with their analogous difficulties, exchanging information about their experiences and communicating via the Internet. He explained that the idea had originated during the Turin event and that they had already been contacted by the community of Mongolian shepherds. This group of nomads travels across the immense Asiatic steppes raising animals (including the extremely rare Przewalski horse, which is on the verge of extinction), for meat is the only source of nourishment in an environment where nothing grows.

I realized that the network I had imagined had already formed without any action from us, and that Terra Madre alone had already encouraged this kind of contact. It is therefore not utopian to think that the various modern means of communication can be put at the service of this idea; indeed, the example of the Sami and the Mongolians may be a practical demonstration of a new way of circulating ideas and giving self-respect to these peoples, who stoically survive in lands where it is truly difficult to live. It is important to help them to have as dignified a life as possible, for they still have much to teach us, as Claude Lévi-Strauss recently pointed out:

> Although such societies are very different from one another, they have in common the fact that they make man a receiving subject and not a master of creation. This is the lesson that ethnology has learned from them, and let us hope that when they come to join the union of nations these societies will maintain their integrity and that we ourselves may be able to learn from their example.[61]

It is significant that these societies had the idea of a post–Terra Madre network without anyone explaining to them why it was necessary.

1. CREATING A NETWORK

The main project is the network itself. In describing food as a *network* of people, places, products, and knowledge (see the dish of pasta with tomato sauce on p. 174), we inevitably feel part of that network, as gastronomes. We belong to a food network, which goes from the global to the particular, and which exists both on a universal and on a local level, both for those who produce and for those who co-produce. At present, many of the nodes that make up this network do not even know that they are connected; they are kept almost entirely separate and do not communicate at all (think of the separation between producers and consumers). The objective is to reactivate the connections, starting with those meeting the gastronome's criteria of quality and then extending the network as far as possible.

The network, as such, is proving to be a potentially revolutionary tool to meet all kinds of needs, from the global fair-trade economy to interest groups on sustainable activities or the defense of civil rights.

According to the prevalent theory, the main characteristics of a network system are its openness and its ability to sustain itself (which makes it more democratic and gives the right value to diversity). Moreover, a network is described in terms of its *intensity* and *extent*. Intensity means that each node or unit of the network must aim to reach and involve a larger number of people in the area where it operates. This will lead to the creation of new nodes. Extent means "expanding the network toward other areas, collaborating in the creation and development of new nodes, increasing the diffusion of the network and reinforcing it as a whole."[62]

The diversities thus become functional, a force for creation and expansion; they increase the common good (which does not mean that everyone has the same aim, but that everyone feels solidarity with and acts for the interests of all), and they guarantee the survival of the system itself.

As we have already mentioned, as applied to the world of food, the network is potentially already in existence, because food is the element *par excellence* that connects people and social groups. But today, unfortunately, this network of food—of food *as* a network—does not work properly, for it has been undermined by elements of distortion (the loss of knowledge and biodiversity, the impossibility of communication, unsustainability) and undemocratic tendencies (the concentration of economic powers and of productive activities, the standardization and homogenization of taste, sensorial impediment). The idea that the gastronome wishes to propose is that the network be reactivated, and at the same time widened and reinforced (in extent and intensity), while preserving respect for gastronomic science, traditional knowledge, and human dignity, according to the new and precise concept of quality. This does not mean, however—and this should be made clear from the outset—that in the name of an aprioristic judgment we must exclude from the system the rest of the world of food, that is to say, all those parts that are not in line with this project, such as much of modern science, industry, and the present systems of distribution. We should, rather, put pressure on such sectors to persuade them to change their strategies and aims, to bring them into line with the new network.

Still on the subject of planning, we must first identify people who can act as "conscious" nodes in the network, then provide services to enable the network to function properly and be characterized by its content. The aim is to protect diversity and set in motion, or place in a dialectical relationship, the content of the nodes. In this way, if it is a good network, it will be able to sustain itself, taking in new subjects, new nodes, and therefore new diversities, which will reinforce it and promote the flow of the whole, generating new and virtuous transformations and growths. The outcome will be true sustainable development, detached from the idea of economic growth at all costs, and connected to the idea of human growth and to the diffusion of a common good—guaranteeing us a rosier future and quality food for all.

To enable me to explain more clearly the project of a virtuous food network, a network which we shall call "gastronomic"—made up of producers, intermediaries, and co-producers—

I trust the reader will excuse my beginning with a personal story, a concrete example from which these considerations originated. It is only an initial idea, and it derives from the first identification of a particular kind of network: the food community network of Terra Madre.

1.1 The Terra Madre experience

I will not dwell too long on the Terra Madre meeting, which took place in Turin at the Palazzo del Lavoro on October 21–23, 2004. There is already plentiful literature and documentation on the subject,[63] and it is not the aim of this book to promote the initiatives of the movement of which I am president. But that idea, that occasion, and the developments that it is generating are an excellent point of departure for a discussion of the "gastronomic network," so a brief history of its aims and a description of the event will be useful.

The basic idea was to bring together a large number of people from all over the world in a single place—important people, the so-called "intellectuals of the earth": farmers, fishermen, nomads, craftsmen, and others engaged in the production or distribution of food that is good, clean, and fair. We drew on the worldwide network of contacts which has been created through the associative international experience of Slow Food, asking our contacts to indicate groups that would be suitable participants in an event of this kind. We called these groups "food communities" (this first step was the basis of the definitions of the various communities that were given in chapter 4); there were about 1,200 of them, and we made arrangements for their representatives, 4,888 people from 130 different countries, to travel to Turin. There, they would find hospitality and an organization that would involve them in discussions called Earth Workshops, which dealt with general themes such as women's work or desertification, and other more specific ones based on the kind of commodity with which the participants were involved—for example wheat, rice, corn, or fruit. That was our way of linking diverse experiences and laying a constructive foundation for an event that would be able to provide a simple (and folkloristic) demonstration and exhibition of cultural diversity.

Each day's work consisted of two general meetings and a series of Earth Workshops: a large amount of information was exchanged at the specialized meetings, but the two general assemblies were particularly moving and occasions of profound significance.

To take a step back, our basic idea was to bring together people who would never otherwise have had the chance to talk to each other, and to invite them to talk about their own simple, everyday (but vitally important) work. The travel expenses of the representatives of communities from the poorer countries, and in general of anyone who had obvious difficulty in traveling, were met by the committee that was formed for the occasion (comprising Slow Food, the Italian Ministry of Agriculture and Forestry, the Piedmontese Regional Authority, and the Turin City Council); hospitality was provided by civic and religious organizations and by the Piedmontese farming community (with an important contribution from Coldiretti), which opened its houses and farms to the representatives.

Paying travel expenses and providing hospitality and bureaucratic assistance was a completely new departure for such "global" events. It is usually only the rich and leisured or institutional and academic representatives who are able to move around the world to attend such events. But here we introduced respect for the right to travel (as a formative experience and as a means of cultural exchange), a sense of hospitality—which is becoming increasingly rare in the modern world but is fortunately still genuinely present in the farming world—and a sense of giving and absolute confidence in the participants' abilities.

To be honest, it was difficult to foresee all the developments of the event, but the idea of creating a network between the "food communities" (at Terra Madre they were primarily "producing communities") and the "gastronomic co-producers" linked by Slow Food was present from the beginning. Significantly, and symbolically, Terra Madre was held simultaneously with the Turin Salone del Gusto, which brought together other producers from all over the world, as well as, more importantly, 170,000 extremely well-informed visitors.

The Terra Madre event generated enthusiasm among the participants, who undoubtedly (the letters that we received after the event confirm this) felt part of that "community of destiny," made up of shared values, which lies at the heart of these ideas. This feeling of belonging certainly continues to live within them now that they have returned to their communities—and now that they have discovered they are not alone. For Terra Madre did not end with the final general assembly; it did not close a circle, but created new perspectives, opened up a whole new world which is finally aware of what it represents.

1.2 The food community

Here, we should insert a methodological note on the meaning of the concept of the "food community" and the way it evolved through the planning and realization of Terra Madre and the desire to give continuity to the event.

The first step was to seek a definition for the individuals who were to be invited to Terra Madre: an eminently practical need. We decided to group them into units which could be represented by their leaders or by the people best able (perhaps for linguistic reasons) to communicate with other people like them. The information we were given indicated a wide variety of social groups: whole villages, clusters of families, small ethnic groups, associations of small producers, autonomous groups involved in alternative distribution, entire sectors that had formed around the new and precise concept of quality. The geographical definition was for the most part fairly narrow, in the sense that the communities belonged to a well-defined and restricted area, but larger geographical areas were also represented (in the case of associations, groups, or productive sectors), in some cases corresponding to an entire nation.

The result was a selection (our search, after the initial phase, was accompanied by spontaneous requests) of about 1,200 communities, represented in Turin by groups whose individual members were able to articulate as effectively as possible the various professions and sensibilities that combined to guarantee the success of a given product.[64] "Food communities" was chosen because it expresses well the characteristics of these heterogeneous groups. All of them are *communities*—either physically identifiable, as in a village, or having shared values and interests, as in a community of destiny—and all of them are engaged, through the protection of seeds, harvesting, agriculture, animal husbandry, fishing, processing, distribution, promotion, education, and other gastronomic activities, in ensuring that a particular *food*, generally produced on a small scale, reaches the person who will eat it. These communities rarely had a strong institutional identity. It should be stressed that we are outside the world of trade unions and political parties and movements: the producing communities of Terra Madre are made up of simple workers, who before the event felt rather alone in the world.

This, then, was the principle that guided the organizers of Terra Madre and that characterized the event itself: the assigning of food communities to interest groups according to the kind of food they produced, the techniques of production that they used, or the common problems that they faced.

The food communities, however, as well as being the thematic and organizational basis of the event, were also a means and an end: they soon emerged as potential units or nodes of a network. The main desire that they expressed during and after the event was that they should keep in touch with one another, in order to exchange ideas and provide mutual support. In reality, therefore, a network was formed the moment the communities were identified and invited to be part of the general project; that project certainly did not stop with the meeting, but still strives to provide tools and services that may lead to other analogous meetings, possibly even wider in scope.

For the aim is to lay the foundations for a coming together, a union with all other gastronomic subjects: beginning with the new co-producing consumers, such as those who are united under the aegis of the Slow Food movement (whose role in this project, it should be emphasized, is mainly that of providing a service), and including chefs, retailers, craftsmen, and small businessmen. The cement of the union must be *gastronomic interest*, animated by the awareness that everyone is experiencing the same community of destiny. It is likely that all these subjects will therefore have the same desire, the same sense of being part of a terrestrial citizenship driving them to behave according to principles that respect quality and all the diversities; most likely, they are also ready to interrelate with each other and with other external subjects (the "virtuous" networks that already exist).

1.3 *The world network of gastronomes*

Let us be clear about one thing: the plan is not to build a network to which we can then attach an ideological label (much less a trademark, new or existing), but to lay the foundations for a network perfectly able to increase in "intensity" and "extent," and in which expansion is guaranteed in proportion to the diversity that it is able to absorb.

The democratic nature of the network is guaranteed by the equal status of all the subjects involved, who are all considered—because they consider themselves to be such—*gastronomes* in equal measure. They belong to different cultures and can have different roles within the world of food. Grouped together are various food communities which contain these kinds of components:

- nodes which correspond to the productive communities;

- groups of co-producers organized, for example, into gastronomic, ecological, and social associations, or linked together for educational purposes or in order to form buying groups;

- the cooks of the world, at all levels, from international celebrities to small street vendors in the remotest parts of the world, or people who cook for their family or community;

- the universities, the science departments that have gastronomic implications, the centers for research into traditional knowledge, and the people who continue those traditions;

- every single citizen who feels part of a "community of destiny" and wants to have influence on the future through food and everything that concerns it.

But democracy is also guaranteed by the sharing of the values that I have described, which are especially well suited to the project because they all have one thing in common: our definitions of "gastronomy" (agriculture, cuisine, et cetera), "quality," "knowledge," "education," and even the various meanings of "community," are all open to *diversity* and have a precise connotation of something local and particular, which is specific to certain geographic areas.

Therefore, like all networks, the worldwide network of gastronomes, as we will call it, is at the same time local and global, diverse and united, concerned with details and with the whole— with food at its center. It is virtuous, in other words it works for creation and not for destruction; it desires to increase the range of sharing and will not generate new divisions. It is a network that can link up with all the other virtuous networks, those which, focused on other specific needs but always open to diversity and to common values for man, tend to counterbalance the damage caused by Edgar Morin's four engines (see p. 000), creating happiness and well-being.

As I write, I am conscious of the fact that the first members of this network (for example the food communities of Terra Madre, or the Slow Food movement) are only a small fraction of humankind. They make no revolutionary claims, and they are not in a hurry. But the political value of the examples conveyed by the network is important to the extent that it sustains itself, grows and establishes relations and alliances with other networks.

This reminds me of an image which an old Piedmontese emigrant (from my own hometown) described to me years ago.

If he were still alive, he would be over a hundred today and, like many Piedmontese, he emigrated in his youth to Argentina. After telling me stories of Buenos Aires in 1908, where the aesthetic canons of the tango were developed, where in some districts people conversed in Piedmontese dialect, and where the migrant communities were based on feelings of solidarity that hardly exist anymore, he added that in the pampas he once saw an invasion of grasshoppers stop a train. The wheels of the train became oily through running over them and spun freely, losing their grip on the rails: insects succeeded in stopping the machine.

We, too, are a very small portion of the human race, like insignificant grasshoppers. The network of gastronomes numbers a couple hundred thousand people today, but it already has shared values which will steadily expand its range, as it links up with the other exponents of virtuous globalization. When we start to lose the feeling of being alone (as the participants in Terra Madre have found out for themselves) and we are able to work in the name of our community of destiny, no business, no change, no machine will be able to stop our quest for happiness. We are like those grasshoppers that stopped the train.

1.4 *How it can work and why it must work*
The *worldwide network of gastronomes* is thus based on ideas, but also has practical implications which enable it to be recognized and to function effectively. Those who wish to promote the network must see themselves as providers of services: that of supplying tools and of stimulating debates, exchanges, and the circulation of knowledge, products, and people.

It goes without saying that when we speak of a network, we must inevitably look to the new communication technologies and the technological resources available to cultures. The Internet is today the greatest tool of global communication and is well suited to the needs of the network of gastronomes: it establishes contact; it facilitates the exchange of information; it can hold files that are freely available to consult with no limitations of space or time; and it makes possible mobilization in real time and the managing of new systems of distribution.

Although it is not an absolute precondition, the computer must be provided as an essential tool, though we must try to avoid its obvious limitations—in particular, the possible difficulty of access in some parts of the world. This is a problem of computer literacy and of infrastructures, which can be solved, if only slowly. While it is true that at present the world is still divided into those who have access to the Internet and those who do not, it is also true that the number of people who have access to it is increasing very rapidly. Satellite and computer technologies will certainly make the Internet available to all, as it potentially already is; in many food communities, even in the most remote and isolated ones, communication via Internet is already a reality. It is not surprising, therefore, that when I visit a village of the Krahô people in Tocantins, central Brazil, I hear the people promise, on my departure, to keep in touch, and proudly offer me a piece of paper with their email address on it.

We must strive to provide resources and to make use of expert advice to devise a computer network that can support the network of gastronomes: a proper service. This may be the form that gives the network recognizability, and therefore identity.

This is an aspect of *planning*, because this is how the network must work; this is the aim of those who, inevitably, must administer it and guarantee the continuity of the whole. The operation of the network will later make possible the implementation of other projects that will proceed alongside the emergence of new alternative values: the concept of products being free in the financial sense; an economy detached from a dependence on money; the economic promotion (which does not mean the monetization) of nonmaterial goods and of specific abilities; innovative and sustainable rules for the distribution of products; an extensive right to mobility; mutual enrichment based on different human experiences; and new dignity for traditional forms of knowledge and for the life of farming communities.

The aim of the network is to make these alternative strands operative, to support them and finance them with specific resources. Each act of planning is part of the whole project of the network, and makes use of it. In the network, the experiences and skills of the participants are modulated in a functional manner, while the cultural diversity within it is exploited in a productive manner. In sum, a new creativity is proposed which looks to the past and to history (including the microhistory of each community, of each person) to demonstrate its modernity, and which looks to the present situation to bring into focus the problems of the earth and of the *stomach*, to guarantee a future which is different from that for which we seem destined.

This is not mere utopia, but political theorization, an intellectual effort to find ways of developing certain human forces which at present are mistreated and undervalued. The network can—and must—work, because it is a means of gradually correcting some macroscopic distortions of our food system and of introducing into the machinery regulating the workings of the world certain values that can be easily translated into everyday practice with the help of the system that we have in mind. The following sections will provide the first examples of this effort to link ideas with their realization and ideals with the functions that they can fulfill if they are included in the worldwide network of gastronomes—which fortunately has already expressed its potential, though only a few years have passed since the first edition of Terra Madre. The network of gastronomes must be able to guarantee the circulation within itself:

- of information, at all more or less virtual levels, by using computers and oral means of communication and by implementing *educational* strategies;

- of *knowledge*, old and new, gastronomic and otherwise;

- of *products*, so that they conform to the new idea of quality and are good for the palate and the mind, sustainable for the earth, and fair because every person's dignity is guaranteed.

- of *people*, because they are the fulcrum of the network, and their mobility, their ability to have direct experiences, to meet other people and to learn from them things that cannot be learned from books are the main conditions that must be fulfilled if this network is to find strength, resources, knowledge, information, and products, and if all humankind is to unite around it.

{**DIARY 15**} SHORT CIRCUIT
SAN FRANCISCO–BAJARDO

In early January, around the Epiphany holiday, it has become a personal tradition for me to spend a few days on the Côte d'Azur with Alberto Capatti and Vittorio Manganelli thinking about and planning the work for the University of Gastronomic Sciences of Pollenzo and Colorno. In January 2004, on my way home from there, following the advice of Slow Food's restaurant guide *Guida delle Osterie d'Italia*, we headed for Bajardo, a tiny village inland from Ventimiglia; we stopped at the Trattoria Armonia, where you feel as if you have gone back in time and rediscovered the ancient flavors of traditional Ligurian cuisine. The road from Ventimiglia is particularly bad, and to make matters worse, halfway along it we ran into a minor snowstorm; but the effort of the journey was amply repaid by the wonderful lunch we were served in this hamlet of a few inhabitants. The onward journey from there was equally eventful: it took us three hours to get home, in the midst of the snow, which continued to fall thickly all afternoon.

Only three days later, I had to fly to San Francisco to participate in the work of the American board of Slow Food, and during a pause in the proceedings I went to one of the most richly stocked record shops I have ever seen: Amoeba Music on Haight Street. My old passion for folk music directed me straight to the relevant shelves, and I came across records from the collection of traditional music recorded by Alan Lomax, the doyen of ethnomusicologists, during his trip to Italy in 1954. Lomax had traveled the world hunting for recordings of folk music, building up an immense archive which is partly preserved at the Smithsonian Institution in Washington, D.C. In the Italian collection, published by Rounder Records, I found a CD of music from Liguria, entitled *Bajardo*. I was astonished. Almost incredulous, I bought the CD and took it to my hotel. I listened to it immediately and learned from the sleeve notes and photographs that it had been recorded in the very village where I had eaten only a few days earlier. I immediately called the trattoria owner in Bajardo, but he knew nothing of this precious recording. I asked him to make inquiries, and sure enough the old people of the village remembered the names of those singers who fifty years earlier had performed for an American visitor. But none of them was still alive; how sad to learn that this memory is preserved in Washington, whereas in Italy the Ligurian Regional Council and the village of Bajardo itself had no idea that these recordings even existed. They were epic ballads, the kind so well described in the nineteenth century by Costantino Nigra, with precious performance techniques such as the Genoese *trallallero*, which is now almost extinct. The songs accompanied rites characteristic of social or festive gatherings that have survived only in the grooves of this record by Lomax, who in 1954, armed with a bag containing a bulky tape recorder, managed to persuade the inhabitants of Bajardo to perform them for him. Lomax was joined on that journey by Diego Carpitella, perhaps the greatest ethnomusicologist that Italy has produced. I could not help wondering whether this science, ethnology, will one day receive the recognition that it deserves.

For we are now in a situation which requires, more than ever before, an emergency ethnology, before too much of Italian history and the history of others is lost. That short circuit between San Francisco and Bajardo was what triggered this train of thought in me—which made me feel the need to document and preserve the characteristic expressions of all the food communities of the world. These expressions are intimately linked with gastronomic culture and, quite apart from their indisputable documentary value, they provide a solid basis both for a future historiography of the new gastronomy and for a better understanding of the food communities with which it interacts.

I think recording, cataloguing, and storing of such information are the duties of the members of the community: it is they who must make sure that they hand down, by any means possible, their songs, stories, rites, habits, and customs.

Indeed, the short circuit between San Francisco and Bajardo reawakened an old passion and the memory of a meeting that was a crucial element in my education and that today impels me to support with even more conviction the idea of this "emergency ethnology."

In 1977, I would never have imagined that five years later my interest would have turned to gastronomic questions. Those were the years when my political and cultural commitment manifested itself in my work in the local cultural association and in the opening of a bookshop at Alba, in the province of Cuneo. It was during that period that I met Nuto Revelli, who had just written his great work, *Il mondo dei vinti* (The World of the Defeated), based on recordings and transcriptions of the oral memories of the farmers of the Cuneo area. This method, and Revelli's sensibility, immediately won me over, especially as during those years my visits to the *osterie* of the Langhe often brought me into contact with the people who were the object of his research. This documentary approach so convinced me that on behalf of the Istituto Ernesto De Martino, I, too, started recording (without even knowing who Lomax was) traditional songs of the *osteria*. After all, these were my people, and if I think today about how much of this culture has disappeared with those last witnesses of it, I am filled with regret, for the work that I began could and should have been far more intensive. That really was a treasure which has now been lost.

But in 1990, I had the opportunity to make use of this experience in my *Atlante delle Grandi Vigne di Langa* (Atlas of the Great Vineyards of Langhe), which was a response to the need to catalogue and describe the great *crus* of Barolo and Barbaresco. The only way of defining the geography of the great wines of southern Piedmont was to draw on the knowledge of the country people and, naturally, on the few specialized studies on the subject: *Monografia sulla viticoltura ed enologia nella provincia di Cuneo* (A Monograph on Viticulture and Enology in the Province of Cuneo) by the agronomist Lorenzo Fantini, published in the late nineteenth century; the study *Sulla delimitazione delle zone a vini tipici* (On the Delimitation of the Growing Areas of Typical Wines) by Ferdinando Vignolo Lutati, published in the 1920s; and *Carta del Barolo* (A Map of Barolo) by Renato Ratti, which dates from the 1970s.

To these basic sources, I added more than five hundred hours of recordings made among the oldest winegrowers and their wives. The extraordinary thing is that in addition to the work on the delimitation of the *crus* (for which the country people's memories of the use made of the grapes of this or that vineyard were indispensable), there emerged a series of testimonies which aptly described the local economy and the winegrowing culture of the early twentieth century. Of all the books published by Slow Food, the *Atlante* is undoubtedly closest to my heart, for even today when I look at the photographed faces and re-read the stories, I realize that those testimonies evoke the former life of country communities which are so different today.

And it was all thanks to the inspiration that Revelli gave me through his incredible work: those words conveyed all the life, the gastronomy, the economy, the culture, the social life of those times—hard times, when the people, amid great privations, were active subjects who contributed to the transformation of the land. I am glad that the *Atlante* has preserved for future generations the difficult life of the land of my birth, a life summed up by a woman of Serralunga d'Alba as follows:

> The sharecroppers' life was hard; the landowners never divided the crops into equal halves, but always gave us a little less. We had no security, and if the landowner sold out, you could find yourself out on the road. On St. Martin's Day you moved to another farm; it was a wretched life.

If there is one thing I feel at this moment, it is a strong desire that Revelli's method should become standard, institutionalized practice. The contribution of the new recording technologies is immense, and the oral history of simple people, their microhistory, has as yet been little explored. When at Terra Madre I saw the faces of the participants and heard their stories, I became even more convinced that the mission of cataloguing was vitally important and that it should be implemented, as I have already said, in the first place by the communities themselves.

Indeed—partly to set an example, and partly because the idea really fascinates me—I immediately set to work in my own town, Bra, where some colleagues and I founded a little historical institute whose purpose is to preserve the memory of Bra and of its inhabitants. The institute continues the small amount of research that has been done on the town's past, and makes video recordings of a large number of elderly people describing their lives and their relationship with the town. The results are published periodically in a journal (*Bra, o della Felicità*, a title devised by the Piedmontese writer Gina Lagorio, a refined intellectual of whom I shall always have a fond memory), and we are building up an archive of the recordings and of all the other material that is being uncovered through the efforts of the local people involved in the initiative. I began in my own backyard, as I hope others will do, and I dream of a worldwide network that will work to create this kind of archive, which with complete systematization will constitute a treasure of inestimable value for future generations and for the new gastronomic science.

....

2. BRINGING ABOUT CULTURAL CHANGE: A HOLISTIC VISION OF THE WORLD OF GASTRONOMES

The main channel of the network of gastronomes is of course that of gastronomy, of food production in the widest possible sense. But if we take into account the arguments outlined above and of the aim of guaranteeing the circulation of knowledge within the network, two other factors immediately come into play: on the one hand, the need to link the gastronomic disciplines in a exchange between the traditional forms of knowledge and modern science, the "dialogue between realms"; and on the other hand, the need, when the network expands and becomes part of a system with other networks, to open our *vision* to a far wider sphere than the gastronomic channel, which is complex enough in itself (see chapter 4).

These factors are not incompatible with the general project of the network; in fact, I am convinced that they are structural and that they can constitute an element of strength and novelty, as well as modernity.

For the "dialogue between realms" finds in the network its greatest potential manifestation: the network includes both the traditional producing communities, with their cultures and their techniques, and, for example, the universities that deal with food production and agriculture, without excluding subjects like anthropology, ethnography, and history.

The same may be said of chefs—the main direct links between production and consumption at the local level—who, thanks to the network, find themselves in the same virtual place as people who, for example, study the modern technologies of nutrition or food processing.

The network of the gastronomes is therefore able to establish an exchange between different realms of knowledge, thus generating new identities, new progress, sustainable innovation, and sufficient communication between the different specializations, which are at present too self-contained or not sufficiently respected by "official" culture.

This dialogue between realms has already been thoroughly defined and discussed by agroecological theory (see chapter 2 and Diary 10), which is based not only on biodiversity but on an active recovery of the traditional forms of knowledge of country people. There is even a gastronomic school, more reflective than some of the others, which understands very well that it must include the study of both the history of peasant nutrition and artisanal culinary traditions, which are the greatest expression of all that constitutes gastronomy.

This dialectical capacity, which can carry out a fruitful task of conservation and enable different forms of knowledge to meet on equal terms in dignity and authoritativeness, must start from a profound cultural change, from an epistemological shift, from a different approach to knowledge.

This change finds its driving ideal in the network, if the latter is initiated, as it logically should be, on the level of respect for all diversities and for the lived experience of peoples, groups, communities, and people who enter the system. As the network expands and intensifies, this change inevitably differentiates the cultural areas of interest and accepts them as active elements of the system itself. To put it more clearly, this is a widening of the vision of the network, a greater consciousness of the complexity that surrounds food, a natural and cultural element, and therefore always placed in a context.

What is needed is what I would call a "holistic" cultural vision for the network of gastronomes: a vision which, in order to redeem gastronomy from the folkloristic sphere to which it has been relegated, holds in equal regard the other aspects of the popular cultures, especially that which is commonly described as "folklore."

2.1 Creating a global cataloguing system for traditional culture
Redefining gastronomy is also an effort to redeem its scientific dignity. Just like the science which we examine in this book, other forms of traditional culture have been relegated to the folkloristic sphere, such as dance, song, oral traditions, architecture, craftwork, and certain productive practices (such as the making of tools). What is the folkloristic sphere? That which pertains to folklore, a manifestation of identity which is redolent of the past, often carrying echoes of hard times; the folkloristic no longer belongs to the people, because the traditions live on only in pageants, parades, and similar reenactments coinciding with festive occasions—such as village fairs—and are no longer everyday practice.

It would be preferable to make these manifestations of cultural identity *part of folklore*, rather than *folkloristic*. By this, I mean that they must belong to the people again, that they must have the chance to survive, or at least to be well known. In those instances where habits and customs have already profoundly changed, active conservation must take place, and wherever the practices are still very present in everyday life, there must be a fruitful relationship of exchange.

The cultural annihilation that has affected the rural world in the last fifty years, and which continues to be perpetrated as the model of agroindustry spreads to new areas of the planet, doesn't just concern food and the environment; the destruction has likewise affected a series of modes of being, ways of communicating and of self-representation that are typical of, and fundamental to, the identity of country people. These modes of being constitute the cultural skeleton of the rural population and contain other forms of knowledge, different from the scientific ones, but no less important.

The idea of a network of gastronomes that neglects to ensure that such manifestations of cultural identity are saved and studied, made alive and functional, their characteristic elements surviving in every detail, would be a contradiction in terms. These manifestations give traditional culture its local specificity, and, like biodiversity and agricultural practices, it is not possible to imagine them detached from the system of food production. It is right that these elements of popular culture should remain an integral part of agricultural systems at the complex local level. They are a structural element of them.

Another task of the network of gastronomes must therefore be that of extending its interests beyond food, seeing productive systems as a unified whole and protecting all diversity with profound respect.

The project, already mentioned in chapter 4, must be to give priority to the urgency of preserving songs, dances, oral traditions, and all the other expressions of identity. The first step toward making it possible for these forms of expression to remain functional to the systems of production that they characterize is to make sure they do not disappear.

The network should also undertake the task of beginning the process of cataloguing all these forms of knowledge: by filming them, transcribing them, and recording them, rather in the manner of the Smithsonian Institution or the Istituto Ernesto De Martino of Sesto Fiorentino, which has worked on Italian traditional music. Today, storage techniques are perfectly adequate for this purpose and also allow more immediate access to their content. We can only imagine what it will mean in a few decades to have such a global storage system at our disposal. If every community undertook to hand down films, interviews with elders, and audio recordings, there would be a corpus of material whose potential in terms of content of traditional knowledge would be enormous.

In conclusion, it will be useful to summarize the reasons why—in addition to the obvious need to preserve traditional knowledge—we must plan the systematic documentation and storage of these characteristic forms of expression, and not only of those relating to food:

- They contain popular knowledge, which has not yet been sufficiently brought into dialogue with the other spheres of knowledge, and this must be saved before it becomes unusable.

- They are the characteristic representation of the communities; they are a reason for pride, but also a key to understanding for anyone from outside who wishes to enter into contact with those communities. Learning them is a form of respect, but also a way of communicating.

- Since they are an integral part of the community's production system, they must inevitably influence it in some way and can help us study it in more detail. They are part of the context, which, as we have seen, is never irrelevant as far as food production is concerned.

- They will be able to guarantee an adequate historiography of the producer communities and of the people in the network, highlighting over the course of the years the most fruitful models of exchange and the solutions to common and analogous problems. At the same time, they will reinforce the "identity" of such forms of knowledge, by which I mean the tangle of roots (see chapter 2) which constantly generates and fuels them. At the moment, this kind of historiography (including the historiography of food) does not have enough material to perform its task effectively (because such material generally derives from the poorer classes, which have few means of self-representation).

2.2 The universities and agroecology

A systematic cataloguing of the forms of knowledge, techniques, folklore, and all the other forms of expression of the food-producing communities is not an end in itself, even though it does constitute a heritage of inestimable value.

Agroecological theory claims to be a science strongly influenced by the traditional knowledge of country people. These forms of knowledge are accorded the status of a science, with the same dignity as all other sciences, because they are the specific result of centuries of development carried out by simple empiricism and by the instinct of adaptation to the environment. The traditional forms of knowledge fit perfectly into the environmental context, and the context (biodiversity, climate, geomorphology) in turn makes it possible to understand fully their motivations and usefulness. It goes without saying that without a context these forms of knowledge lose strength, meaning, and the possibility of application. From the perspective of conservation, traditional forms of knowledge are a precious resource, and their maintenance, study, and reorganization help to create the conditions for sustainable development.

But if we accept the importance of the environmental context, we must accept the importance of the social context, too. These same forms of knowledge that make it possible to cultivate and produce are equally connected in a system of rites, beliefs, cosmology, habits, and customs, as well as in oral, artistic, and technological forms of expression. So it is clear that in order to operate in the network, to keep it active, we must take into account those forms of knowledge that concern the social life of the communities. The entire context in which they exist must be saved in order to continue a harmonious line of development; instead, this harmony has been brusquely interrupted by the introduction of unsustainable techniques, which are too invasive and disrespectful of what exists.

Therefore, alongside the work of cataloguing, the overall project must involve the development of the catalogue, the maintenance of its operation, the study of its functional value to the productive system, and of its educational implications.

In view of the far-sightedness with which traditional agroecology is imbued, it will perhaps be advisable to link those who are engaged in cataloguing traditional knowledge (the communities themselves, one hopes) with those who are engaged in agroecology and development, so that the latter can both benefit from the catalogue and contribute to it, highlighting the links between folklore and small-scale agricultural activity, in the name of that holistic vision, of that cultural change which is the second project of the network.

The most effective way to start off this virtuous process is, in my view, to rejuvenate the academic culture in these areas, identifying the scholars most sensitive to it and including them in the network. I would like to see the creation of entire university departments dedicated to traditional agroecology, where the anthropological and ethnographic studies—with the support of the great multimedia catalogue of the network—are an integral part of the educational and research process.

Planning in this case therefore strongly involves the academic world and the scholars of these disciplines, who must be urged not to become closed within their own specializations, but to open up to other disciplines in order to further investigate the existing complexity. It is up to the scholars to reinterpret, to redefine, the values of the traditional cultures, which both in the West and in the developing countries are undergoing attacks and threats of every kind and disappearing at an unimaginable speed. Just think how many languages, how many dialects are dying out or have died out during the last few years: this is just one of the many indexes of a disappearance of identity, and it makes one fear the cultural homogenization toward which we are hurtling with such speed in Morin's unsustainable "four-engined spaceship" (which I spoke about on page 17).

2.3 A "holistic" network of knowledge
Broadening our cultural and operative vision, making it virtually "holistic," entails in the first place the defense of diversity and complexity, linking them in a network, making them functional to the project of enabling the earth to regain, through the systems of food production, the *right rhythm.*

Cataloguing the traditional forms of knowledge is an act of conservation and respect; embarking on the multidisciplinary study of them (from agriculture to song) represents an effort to regard problems from the widest and most all-embracing point of view possible. As gastronomic science teaches us, it takes many lenses to understand systems with so many different inputs. One has to superimpose them, find analogies, connections between different "realms," in a kind of interpretative schema which helps decipher the complexity by bringing about a meeting between the two axes on which modern science and traditional knowledge stand, as well as various levels of particularity and generality (local/global, specialist/holistic).

All this, linked up in a network, generates a complexity which is undoubtedly difficult to administer, but let us remember that the network does not in fact need to be administered. All one has to do is to guarantee its functioning so that it will be understood as clearly as possible, thus facilitating the direction of any action that people may wish to take.

Since this complexity is in fact the network itself, in this way, by thriving on diversity on various levels, it cannot fail to guarantee its own sustainable functioning. The holistic vision of traditional and gastronomic culture is in this sense an integral part of a very ambitious project.

{**DIARY 16**} CHIAPAS, ROCKEFELLER, AND
THE SMALL FARMERS OF PUGLIA

In many years of meetings with the food communities, I have constantly found myself coming up against inconsistencies in the market which cause enormous problems for farmers, whether in the Western world or in the developing countries. I have seen how the two extremes of what is commonly called the food chain are constantly penalized: on the one hand, the farmers, on the other, the consumers—producers and co-producers who have to cope with situations which border on the paradoxical.

For example, in 2001 in Mexico, the impoverished farmers of the Los Altos area in Chiapas were faced with a series of terrible problems connected with the production of their indigenous varieties of corn.

Corn originated in Mexico. The Maya believed that mankind had developed from a corn cob, and even today in the region of Montezuma there are hundreds of varieties of this product. What is astonishing, however, is that almost 40 percent of the corn that is consumed in Mexico is imported from the United States. What's more, numerous native Mexican varieties have been patented in the United States, becoming in effect an American agroindustrial product.

It was almost natural that the farmers of Los Altos—without knowing how to read and write, and without ever having participated in the worldwide debate on globalization—should begin to wonder why they could find only the white variety of corn at the market, and U.S.-made white corn flour, even though they themselves usually grew red, black, or yellow corn. They couldn't understand, either, why the *coyotes* (the commercial intermediaries) paid them 1.5 pesos a kilo for the surplus from their harvest, and yet when they needed corn because the harvest had been poor, the *coyotes* demanded 6 pesos—for a different and inferior variety.

It was necessary to intervene in some way, so it was decided to form a Presidium with the Los Altos farmers to safeguard their four main native varieties and to remedy the unfair distortions of the market. The meetings seemed interminable, with translations from Italian into Spanish and then into their indigenous language, *tzotzil.* Their community decision-making process is as directly democratic as one could possibly imagine; everyone can and must participate. In the end, they accepted a small initial amount of financial support to help them change their system and run it, thus protecting their own varieties, but above all so that they could earn more and spend less.

The financial support, through training courses with local agronomists, served to reconstruct the *milpa* (a small, family-based, mixed-crop farming unit to which agroecological theory attaches great importance). The *milpa* is ideal for family self-sufficiency and for environmental conservation, but is strongly opposed by the *coyotes,* who favor the monoculture. Authorization was given for genetic research on behalf of the local farmers in order to give them exclusive rights to the genetic heritage of native corn, thus eliminating the danger of piracy which they so much feared, having already suffered from it in the past. But more than anything else, a simple but brilliant solution was found to their commercial problems: the production chain between the communities was closed, eliminating the intermediaries and reconstructing an internal market thanks to a collective brand and an official price—stable for everyone—of about 4 pesos. Anyone who had an excess to sell would earn 4 instead of 1.5 pesos, and anyone who had to buy corn to eat because the harvest had failed would spend 4 pesos instead of 6.

From this simple example, one can understand how the shortening of a food-and-agriculture chain can bring benefits both to the initial seller and to the final buyer (the farmers and the co-producers), but unfortunately we are far from arriving at a fruitful replanning of the trading and distribution systems. And the problem also afflicts the rich areas of the world.

In July 2005, in Italy, while the question of the farmers of Puglia who were underpaid for the production of tomatoes and grapes was being expressed with passion, and in some cases with violence (the protests were later calmed by the decision to pay a political, subsidized price and send grape juice to developing countries as humanitarian aid), I had the privilege to meet David Rockefeller, who at the venerable age of ninety is the last living child of the magnate John D. Rockefeller, Jr. He is a remarkable character: his physical condition is exceptional for a man of his age, but above all he shows an intellectual curiosity that would put many forty year olds to shame. I met him in his New York office, after having visited his model farm, Stone Barns, about a hundred kilometers to the north, in the valley of the Hudson River. The history of the farm dates from the late nineteenth century, when the head of the family, David's grandfather, John D. senior, wanted a country estate to farm dairy cows, because he wanted to drink fresh milk every morning. Since that time, when young David used to spend his summers in the country, the farm might have gone bankrupt had it not been for the initiative of David's late wife, Peggy, a great enthusiast of the agricultural life and the countryside, who completely revived Stone Barns. In 1996, as a tribute to his wife, David decided to give the family farm a new lease on life and made it into an example of sustainable farming and high-quality produce, in contrast to the prevailing emphasis in the American rural sector, which leaves much to be desired in this respect.

Today, it is delightful to visit the handsome buildings of Stone Barns and the surrounding fields, the half-acre greenhouse which produces excellent organic vegetables all year round, and the cattle sheds set in a relaxed environment. It is not just a philanthropic venture, however, but has been planned to be fully profitable while respecting all the criteria of sustainability. Everything is recycled, and so much compost is produced that it cannot all be used on the farm, and so they must sell it. The variety of produce is great, ranging from all sorts of vegetables to the main traditional stock breeds. The farm also carries out an intense educational program, with New York schools coming to visit almost in a continual cycle.

I was struck by the fact that in order to make perfectly profitable this effort to produce food in a manner that was good, clean, and fair, they had resorted to autonomous distribution systems. For the fruit of this work—which employs many young farm workers with great ideas for the future—is either sold through a CSA (Community-Supported Agriculture, see pp. 173–174) to seventy member families or at farmers' markets in nearby towns. Most of the produce, however, goes to the two restaurants affiliated with the farm, both called Blue Hill: one is on the farm itself and the other in Manhattan. In total, the two Blue Hills serve 1,500 meals a day, always using fresh produce which can be reliably traced to its source, and prepared under the guidance of the talented young chef Dan Barber.

The project works wonderfully well—it is a prototype that should be replicated elsewhere. This association between farm, restaurant, the public, and young farm workers, with its focus on sustainability and quality, is an extremely modern production model, which is profitable and completely multifunctional. It shows that this approach can work, and there is a real alternative to traditional agribusiness on an industrial scale, with its unsustainable model of selling and distributing food.

I think of the absurdity of farmers demonstrating in Puglia because their standardized, low-quality produce wasn't bought by a mass-distribution system already flooded by overproduction in other areas (some of it perhaps from abroad, where the vegetables and fruit ripen earlier and are cheap). When angry protests broke out because a whole year's profits were in danger of being lost, the government was forced to pay the farmers subsidies, thereby distorting the market, while the surplus was sent to poor countries in the form of humanitarian aid, undermining those countries' fragile markets and their already problematic and meager production. Instead, what we must do is redefine the distribution systems, shorten the chains, and take our example from model firms like Stone Barns or from small projects of local direct trade, as in Chiapas.

If they were to emphasize quality and variety—rather than quantity, as demanded by the industrial food distribution system—and at the same time develop alternative and local markets, for whom added values such as quality, purity, and justice would be worth the price of a product, I am sure that the farmers of Puglia could avoid situations such as that of the summer of 2005 and could finally have a real chance to improve their lot.

3. CREATING A FAIR AND SUSTAINABLE FOOD DISTRIBUTION SYSTEM

One of the present drawbacks of the agricultural system, both at the global and at the local level, is that of the distribution systems. The last fifty years have seen not only the industrialization and consequent centralization of agriculture (read, specialization by geographical areas) and mass exodus from rural areas, but also the perfecting and improvement of food conservation techniques. Today, a particular food can easily travel from one side of the globe to the other, and in many cases this is actually indispensable, if one thinks of products of mass consumption such as tea, coffee, or cocoa, which are consumed globally but can be grown only in certain areas, or of the provision of food for those large sections of the world population (about half of it) who live in urban areas where food is more difficult to produce. However, with transport and preservation so easy and widespread in the food industry, farmers in many areas have had to abandon crops in the face of a flood of outside competition. Natural selection has been replaced with industrial methods that are homogenizing and damaging to biodiversity. The volume of transportation in the industry has soared, although the distance traveled by a food item is almost never reflected in its final price, and this overall increase in transportation has had a devastating impact on the environment.

Moreover, the forming of a global distribution system, dominated by a few big operators who draw strength from their financial structure and supranational operations (although there are plenty of smaller operators, too), has filled the production chain with innumerable intermediaries, thus helping to increase even further the distance between producer and consumer.

Our proposed counterbalance to this distance is, of course, the network of gastronomes and the figure of the co-producer. But the problems posed by this long chain of intermediaries go beyond that of the distance (physical or cultural) between the two ends of the chain. Rather, the graver concern lies in matters of economics, ecology, and social justice.

Take the case of the *coyote* (the first intermediary for Latin American farmers who live far from the centers of population but who produce crops for the mass market): the *coyote* exploits the work of the farmers, who are often deep in debt and suffer from the fluctuating performance of their monoculture crop on the world market. And then there is the Italian example, where farmers faced derisory prices on the wholesale market for goods that netted exceptionally high prices on the retail market. Such distribution practices can be shamefully unjust, as when producers are suddenly excluded from the channels of distribution because of a fluctuation in the price of coffee or cocoa on the world stock market, or they can be almost comic—though no less significant—as in the case of the "Dutch" tulip bulbs in the greenhouses of Costigliole d'Asti (see Diary 1).

The problem of the reorganization of food distribution is therefore of crucial importance; it is one of the essential tasks if we are to give back to the agricultural system the characteristics of the good, clean, and fair, which are being demanded by the gastronomes, producers, and co-producers of the whole world.

Once again, it is not a question of completely rejecting the present system or of repudiating the figure of the trader or the role of trade. Rather, it is a question of exploiting the system's potential, as in the "dialogue between realms," though in awareness of the limitations with which it is confronted and introducing the new concept of sustainable quality as an essential prerequisite to any operation.

3.1 Giving new meaning to trade

Jean-Anthelme Brillat-Savarin, in his *Physiologie du goût*, maintained that "gastronomy belongs to trade, because of its search for the means of buying at the best possible price that which it consumes and of selling at the highest possible profit that which it puts on sale." It is true that these are the principles that govern trade: buying and selling at prices that allow the biggest possible profit. A trader is successful to the extent that he succeeds in carrying out the transaction to his greatest advantage. In light of what has been said so far, however, I believe that this rule needs to be reconsidered today: the utilitarian and individualistic spirit of the trader, which has profited him for centuries, must be corrected in a more *altruistic* direction, or at least in a *communitarian* direction. And this, it should be noted, must be done in the interest of the traders themselves, who are not excluded from the "community of destiny" that concerns us all without distinction.

In the food sector, the refinement of the techniques for "buying at the best possible price" and selling at the highest possible profit has led to a complete domination by trade. The increasingly centralized systems of distribution are no longer respectful of the dignity of the producing communities and of the co-producing consumers. Even the trader's role loses all dignity, reducing the value of food to its mere monetary value, devoid of the many connotations for which I am arguing in this book.

But most of all, this conception of trade in effect excludes from the circuit the highest-quality producers, who find themselves outcasts with no market at all for their wares or, in the more fortunate cases, a market described as "niche"—that is to say, an elitist, exclusive outlet incapable of generating real wealth and development. Reevaluating trade also means rejecting that continual refrain that the gastronome is always having to cope with: "Quality is expensive, it costs too much, it is not democratic." Reevaluating trade means in the first place involving the traders themselves in the recovery of the nobility of their art, so as to place it in some degree at the service of the community and the network, participating in the project for a new distribution system.

The traders would have to recognize the rights of the producing communities and of the co-producers. As it stands, all those who are conscious gastronomes, united in their efforts to achieve a better system and a virtuous network, are excluded from the system—whereas in fact they can and must continue to play a crucial role. For his part, the trader must be able to turn himself into a vehicle of information, as well as of products and money. He must guarantee the transparency of the chain, limiting himself in his speculation and applying the principles of "quality" himself. Within this new *gastronomic* distribution network, the trader must share the values of the network so as not to be considered stubbornly extraneous to it and repaid in the same coin that he is currently giving to the communities and the co-producers: exclusion. At present, the commercial network too often stifles information about food; as well as tilting the food economy in its favor, it does not communicate with the subjects with which it has to deal, taking care to keep them well apart. But the trader is a *channel* along which information about food must travel. I am thinking of what used to happen at the village store or during bargaining at the local market: the trader described the product, provided information about its provenance, its characteristics, and the original human and productive factors. From here, it is only a short step to the defense of these little shops or other forms of direct trade, face to face. This, too, will be a task for the network.

We must provide a basis for the traders themselves to begin to think about a new way of trading, a healthy way to guarantee dignity to all, where "the best possible price" and "the highest possible profit" take on new meanings; where it is not just money that counts, but social justice, respect for the environment, and, of course, respect for those who produce and for those who eat and put their trust in them. Trade must be a noble art at the service of the community, and the process will be complete when the rights to equity and fairness are also shared by those who trade, in the sense that they, too, will be able to appeal to them in the same way as the producing communities and the co-producers do.

If the network of gastronomes can respond to these needs and can involve and educate those who practice a new kind of trade (they are, after all, indispensable), its expansion will immediately cross the path of those who are already experimenting with alternative forms of trade (such as fair trade) and other networks which do not yet feel that they are "gastronomic" but which have made important experiments in new forms of commercialization.

The gastronome who joins in the network, therefore, accepts Brillat-Savarin's definition of trade but is immediately able to make his own distinctions and qualifications. These will be the basis for a food distribution system that is able to exchange knowledge and values between its various components.

3.2 Limiting intermediation

While giving due consideration to the value of trade, its role, and the rules that it must impose on itself to give and acquire dignity, in the planning of new networks what emerges clearly is that intermediation must be limited as much as possible. That is obvious both if we are to succeed in accomplishing the cultural and political project of creating numerous "new gastronomes," and if we are to eliminate the economic injustices which cause many other problems (it is a far from ridiculous theory, for example, that the main cause of the problem of hunger in the world is the global system of food distribution).

Limiting intermediation means in the first place *shortening* the chain along which a product passes from the field to the table. A new start must be grounded on a healthy localism for all those kinds of food which can be grown, raised, and processed near their areas of consumption. Where is the sense in making vegetables, fruit, and meat travel across continents if they can be (and they almost always can) produced locally? Local food has the advantages of freshness, of a greater preservation of flavor in its journey to the table (many "export" varieties have been selected to meet criteria of preservation and resistance to travel, neglecting crucial gastronomic factors such as goodness and taste), and respect for certain criteria of sustainability. For example, with small local productions, the use of chemicals can be very limited, the produce does not travel and therefore does not pollute, and rural areas are kept alive with a native and variegated production (urban purchasing groups are an excellent way of connecting the city to the *living* countryside).

One of the first advantages of this localism is a significant reduction in speculative intermediation, for if the product has a shorter distance to travel, it is almost obvious that it will pass through fewer hands (and fewer increments to the final price).

I find it paradoxical that near my hometown there is a supermarket located in the middle of what is commonly known as Italy's "garden state": here, many excellent varieties of fruit and vegetables are grown which can be bought directly from the producers or at the weekly markets in town, but many of my fellow townspeople prefer the absurd practice of going to the above-mentioned supermarket and buying, perhaps imported from Chile, the same kind of vegetable which they could find almost on their own doorstep. They pay a higher price and get less enjoyment (for those vegetables cannot compete in taste with a freshly picked product and a good native variety) buying a product which has further polluted its land of origin and the whole earth by its intercontinental journey. What is more, in the making of that product it is likely that somebody's work has been exploited, and that biodiversity has been sacrificed to set up industrial monocultures suitable for export. I cannot see much sense in all this.

The task of the network of gastronomes must therefore be to encourage the circulation of goods and products inside the network, in the most sustainable manner possible, respecting the dignity and gratification of those who produce, and emphasizing a concern for quality among all participants. A network of this kind will have the aim of limiting any intermediate commercial shipments that are unnecessary or unsustainable, as well as guaranteeing control of prices to keep them equitable both for sellers and buyers.

In this way, real control over the chain is given back to the producers and the co-producers, to the food communities, who will ensure that the necessary information is circulated together with the products. Thus, we will be able to avoid the situation, so common at the moment, where information and profits are concentrated in the hands of a few subjects. For in this scenario, the traders, simply by distributing the food, have more power and control than those who work in the fields and those who consume, both of whom end up completely cut off from the chain.

The simple rule to follow in order to circulate products in the network is to make food travel as short a distance as possible.

By applying a principle of local adaptation, one can begin with the satisfaction of local demand and then gradually expand when quantity, quality, and the prices of products allow it—without renouncing trade and always respecting the limit of sustainability, or that common sense which I mentioned in chapter 3.

3.3 Putting new elements of evaluation into the commercial circuit

Often the long journey traveled by a product makes it possible for it to be consumed even out of season. This, in my opinion, is not acceptable, because it does not conform to the criterion of naturalness; it certainly increases the number of intermediations a product goes through, not to mention lengthening and centralizing the commercial food chain. Unfortunately, to argue that this kind of trade should not exist is rather utopian, given the potential of the products and the tendency (temptation) toward diversification of his own table that every gastronome has. Here, too, I would recommend common sense, a fair evaluation of the process, and, if I may say so, a sensitivity toward restraint which is part of that honest sobriety I will discuss later and which must be one of the characteristics of the good gastronome.

But the concept of the traveling product is not to be rejected absolutely. In many cases, journeys are necessary; in others, they are simply tolerable because (as in the case of transport by sea) they are not very pollutant and they might even, if the commercial system is equitable, provide important economic opportunities for the producing communities.

From the point of view of transport, a possible idea (as far as the network is concerned at first, but extendable to the whole distribution sector through incentives, taxation, and restrictive laws) would be to introduce a concept similar to that calculated by the researchers Tim Lang and Jules Pretty: food miles (see chapter 3). These comprise the calculation of the environmental costs and of all other "negative externalities" related to the commercial journey that a product faces. They are an important index of sustainability and, to make a practical suggestion, the network of gastronomes could start to indicate them on the label (not only the place of production, but the various means of transport used) and to monetize (for example with a supplementary price) any environmental cost that may be involved.

I am convinced that this form of economic redistribution, this way of conveying useful information, would be a "natural" factor inciting the network system and the general system toward a healthier and fairer localism. By quantifying the number of intermediations and revalorizing trade with new responsibilities, food miles would make prices more transparent—and the buying of an unsustainable product would be a far more considered act than it is today. The system would be redistributed over a production chain that has expanded from the local to the global, satisfying in the first place the needs of the local population and then, if possible (bearing in mind the quantities, the characteristics of the product, and sustainability), those of other communities not easily able to obtain the products in question.

Such a system would provide an incentive to development based on self-sufficiency in the poorer areas of the world and would adjust in a sustainable way—but perhaps it is better to say in a *gastronomic* way, considering all aspects of quality—the balance of consumption in the richer areas.

*3.4 How can the project work? Nodes, communities, chefs,
     gastronomes, and a stock of products*
A project of alternative distribution as I have described it in the preceding sections must rely on the network: it is an essential working project for the new gastronomes. Few intermediaries, a new kind of trade, a preference for consumption at a local level, the introduction of informative elements such as food miles: all of this would find a very fertile terrain in which to spread, at the same time exchanging influences with already existing networks, such as fair trade, that seek to practice systems of sustainable distribution.

But for a project, principles are not enough: one must also think about what to do in practical terms. It is difficult to rely on existing distribution systems, though it is true that some are indeed more sensitive to the themes of sustainability and local consumption. I think we must do our best to become *active subjects* of this distribution: using all possible channels, starting with the basic nodes of the network—the communities—which may be both productive and distributive units, and carrying out a direct exchange with other communities in the network. From this point of view, too, we will need a service structure whose purpose is to make transport as easy and sustainable as possible, making use of traders who renounce simple utilitarianism and themselves become bearers of shared values and controllers of the process.

It is not only the producing communities, the traders, and the co-producers who must work together: all the other subjects can make their contributions. Starting with the chefs, for example, the people who are most active in the direct search for good (and one presumes, clean and fair) products, who often have preferential channels of communication with the communities and the individual producers. Their experience can be a driving force and an excellent point of departure for reflection on distribution systems. If they put themselves at the service of the network, the network could only gain. Moreover, the promotional value of the use of such products in their restaurants is unrivalled, especially as it is generally accompanied by correct information about provenance and mode of use. On the part of the chefs who enter the network of new gastronomes, a precise commitment to the *adoption* of products of food communities near and far (respecting the criteria of sustainability) is another vital step, given their prominence and the new functions that they are assuming on the global gastronomic scene. We must free chefs from the burden and the game-playing of the media circus, of the competition for points in the guidebooks, whose hierarchy of stars pays little attention to the role of the food system, despite its relevance for the future of the restaurant business. It is in the chefs' interest to take on this responsibility, and they should draw full advantage from their gesture, aware of their role as custodians of culinary knowledge and of the best uses of good, clean, and fair products.

The co-producers themselves, formerly mere "consumers," are also called upon to make a significant contribution, now that they know how best to orient their choices, how to be aware in selecting products, and how they might help fulfill their desire to bring producers nearer in all senses. In this way, the co-producer becomes precisely that: he studies alternative systems, seeks the nearest quality products, promotes the work of the communities, even ones remote from him but needing support. The *co-producing gastronome*, with his commitment to education, to the preservation of knowledge and forms of production, with his search for quality and his sense of community, is another fundamental element in this virtuous distribution network.

The network of new gastronomes, basing itself on an exchange of experience and information, can find the best way to *make products circulate*. Equipping the food-producing units and communities for selling is a fundamental step, for it will be necessary to activate all possible channels for direct trading of products. An idea that might make this work a little easier would be to publish (preferably online) a directory containing the characteristics of the products, their location, the names and contact details of the producers, guidance for sustainable purchasing, and the prices.

The *directory* could be organized like a normal hypertext database, with many possible search methods (according to criteria of geography, sustainability, need for support on the part of the community, possibility of buying groups, as well as all the other basic search methods, such as by producer name). Fields of the database would include all the values and information most suited to the new forms of distribution that we hope to introduce.

In this way, the producing and co-producing communities would be close to each other at a virtual level (potential food communities in cyberspace), able to contact each other directly or through a commercial channel that for once does not completely bypass them. They could create new alliances and new chains, in which intermediation—not speculative but working in the interests of common growth—would be guaranteed by the producing communities themselves or by traders respectful of the rights of all.

To redesign food distribution in this way would, moreover, be to adjust its balance in an *equitable* direction, dealing even with very serious problems, such as malnutrition, in a more constructive manner—for example through the revival of agricultural systems where they have disappeared. Giving the poorest communities the incentive to join the network and implement a new agriculture (ecological and small-scale), whose purpose is to satisfy the community's most immediate subsistence needs, is perhaps better than salving one's conscience by sending them free food aid. Such charitable handouts are often only a way of solving the problem of what to do with the surpluses of subsidized agriculture in the rich areas; as such, they represent a forced introduction into the poor areas, outside the laws of the market, of products without a price, thereby undermining the existing resources of the local markets and all desire to construct a real model of sustainable development.

Instead, in emergency cases such as malnutrition or natural disaster, it would be the network that would activate itself, responding to the needs of the communities connected with it, while remaining careful at the same time not to introduce excessive distortions into the system, always conforming to values of free giving and without any immediate obligation to receive anything in exchange. Such, in essence, are the values that should eventually characterize the whole network, reversing the utilitarian logic that currently dominates our markets and all the systems of production. Put simply: better a high level of Gross Domestic Happiness than a high level of Gross Domestic Product.

When I was a child, it was the custom in my family to invite members of the local community who lived in poverty to lunch at religious holidays. The practice was so natural to my mother that it never occurred to me to wonder about the reason for these curious acts of hospitality.

In fact, I think my mother had adopted the habit from the peasant world into which she was born: it was a spirit of generosity to others which, as I later learned from friends of mine who were experts on rural Italian society, was the norm. In the Piedmontese countryside, it was common practice to leave an empty place at the patriarchal table, ready for any eventuality and reserved for a guest.

These "guests" were wayfarers, people who roamed the countryside living on their wits—beggars, destitutes, people who had fallen on hard times for health or financial reasons. The empty place was also next to the man of the house; it didn't matter whether the "guests" were shabbily dressed or even bad-smelling. In all this, it is true that there is much of Christian culture, which is deeply rooted in the Italian countryside—it was important to show that you could be a good Samaritan—but I think there is actually something more, something profoundly ingrained in the country life.

I had confirmation of this when I interviewed the poet Wendell Berry for a dialogue published in the cultural pages of *La Stampa*, and we turned to the subject of the economy of rural communities. He explained to me that in order to make a local economy work well, one must first think about subsistence and then, if there is any surplus, "use it for charitable work or trade." This seemed to me a rather idealistic idea, but Berry persisted:

> In the past, before agriculture was so industrialized, before we had all these tools to reduce the workload, we did our duty in our families and exchanged work with

our neighbors. The rule was that no one stopped working until everyone else had finished their harvest. I knew
people who were proud of having worked in all the farms
of the area without ever receiving a penny. This is not
capitalism; at most it can be seen as a strange form of
investment: investing in the body of the community.[65]

Indeed, when I worked on my collections of interviews for the *Atlante delle grandi vigne di Langa*, the
words of the old country people always expressed this
aspect of rural society, which was sincerely imbued with a
sense of generosity and readiness to give freely, without
expecting anything in exchange. I remember in particular
one woman, a small trader, who told me: "We used to help
each other; I remember there was a family of twelve people and the mother was sick: so we, the women of the
other families, did her washing and then we all cooked
lunch together."[66]

That place at the table at Christmas and Easter was a
legacy of that culture, in which people were always ready
for mutual help with food and work. I am increasingly convinced that these forms of generosity were not merely dictated by a sort of peasant morality, that they were not just a
sort of religious precept that one had to obey, but that they
were an integral part of the economy of those communities.

Generosity as an economic form: it was a way of cop-
ing with social positions of poverty, with forms of hardship,
and it had a precise meaning. As Berry said, it was a form
of investment. Nowadays, the order of values is the exact
opposite. I don't want to sing the praises of the old days
(for, apart from anything else, poverty was much more
common in those days), but I do think that if I look at the
present situation with the same pragmatism with which, in
recent years, I evaluated those extra places at my table as
economic acts, I would be firmly convinced that there is
still a great need for such acts—for new and old forms of
rustic generosity.

4.CREATING A NEW SYSTEM OF VALUES FOR THE NETWORK OF GASTRONOMES

One of the fundamental characteristics of the network of gastronomes is its *humanity*. This humanity can be capitalized in a practical sense, in the first place by promoting the free circulation of people within the network, restoring to travel its irreplaceable educational function as a means of *actually* bringing into contact with one another people who belong to different communities and who therefore represent different identities. The creative force of diversity is achieved through contact, not only virtual (however indispensable that is in our case), but also physical, which requires among other things a continual exercise of the senses and the intellect in order to make fruitful exchanges.

Individualism, egoism, and the economic advantages gained through politics or through forms of old or new colonialism are difficult to uproot from the minds of those who practice these "anti-values" as a strategy of domination and as their only form of the search for happiness. I believe that meeting, traveling, and having direct and profound contact with other cultures is the best way to spread a new common way of thinking. But in order for people to get to know each other, it is necessary that they have, in addition to being able to actually meet, a predisposition to welcome, to discover, to share, to feel the joy of life. Is it utopian to think of a world where hospitality is a shared value as it was in the countryside years ago, when even the poorest family always had a place reserved for a wayfarer or a beggar? Apart from the fact that I am convinced that he who sows utopia will reap reality, I am certainly convinced that a predisposition for giving freely can be very realistic if one begins to think that this predisposition, like other values, has an economic meaning, even if that meaning is not monetizable. What I mean is this: who gets rich in this world? How valuable is the traditional *knowledge* of the producing communities that are disappearing? How valuable are the acts of conservation operated by those who, simply by their work, succeed in producing in a sustainable way, in preserving the good, clean, and fair that exists in the world?

How valuable is a present, a bed to sleep in, an invitation to a table, a sharing of one's own identity, and an openness to those of others?

Just as I have proposed that we put on the balance sheet the environmental costs, which are so difficult to quantify, I want analogously to propose the project of a network which gives economic weight to the important values that it carries within it—not translating them into money, nor trying to make a profit from them, but inserting them in a logic of exchange, or rather in a logic of *giving freely* where there is no utilitarian exchange, but a mutual giving of knowledge, hospitality, opportunities, tastes, visions of the world, and educational elements. It is a question of giving without asking, but in the certainty that one will receive something in exchange because we are all on the same level, with the same dignity and the same predisposition to make others grow, in an awareness of the *limits,* and with a commitment not to exceed them merely to enrich oneself with money and lose in *humanity.*

4.1 The value of travel

No system of transmitting knowledge within the network can ever replace direct contact. As gastronomic science teaches us, the exercise of one's own sensoriality, trying, tasting, contact with producers and with chefs, is the best way of learning how to interpret reality. To achieve this form of learning, it is necessary to *move,* to meet people, to experience other territories and other tables. If we apply this conviction to the network, it is vital to guarantee the circulation within it of people, from one side of the globe to the other, without distinction and without restriction. The *right to travel* becomes fundamental, a premise on which to base cultural growth and the self-nourishment of the network of gastronomes.

The value of Terra Madre, apart from all other considerations, was partly that of travel, of giving the chance to travel to people (the "intellectuals of the earth") who had never been able to leave their own villages, their own territories, their own regions, to see a section of the world, in a place where they were welcomed by other country dwellers and people engaged in food production and where they would meet five thousand other men and women who worked on the same front as they. In fact, the idea is more revolutionary than it might seem. How many people of the rich West travel in order to solve the problems of those who are in difficulty? And how much does this cost? I am not referring only to a missionary logic, but also to someone who has fewer proselytizing aims and perhaps at most has a sacred respect for the environmental and cultural systems in which he goes to operate.

The educational value of travel has no equal in a world—that of food production based on traditional knowledge—where knowledge is handed down in a direct manner supported by empirical demonstration, trial, and work itself. The image of thousands of representatives of the food communities traveling the world and receiving hospitality from other communities may worry those who have an interest in maintaining the present situation. The diffusion of knowledge achieved in this way could be dramatic; it could open the minds of intelligent people who today are bowed down by the sheer effort of surviving and of producing, without any gratification, *our food*. People who feel alone and abandoned, left culpably devoid of any opportunity to *enrich themselves* from the cultural point of view, suddenly offered the chance to come into contact with a network that shares their efforts and ideas. These are people who are tempted to abandon their invaluable work: but I saw new hope in the eyes of those who participated in Terra Madre, and this has been confirmed by the news I received once they returned to their communities. And this hope would have been born even without the discussions during Terra Madre. All it took was travel, the chance to meet other people, and pride in feeling important with their own knowledge and products. The anxiety to make themselves known, which was the most common feeling among the participants during the event, was the clearest proof of this. These people have much to say and much to give; we must provide them with the opportunity to do so.

At the planning level, it is not a question of inventing methods of exchange, cultural formats, or particular theories; all we need to do is make it possible for these people to travel, to help them to do so. They will do the rest. We must, in the perspective of a "dialogue between realms," in the conviction of the value of traditional knowledge and of the humanity which these people convey, encourage a *faith* in them and in their potential, and especially the potential of the younger generation.

The most deserving of the young people (according to criteria such as a passion for their work, their aspirations and plans, and even their idealism) should be able to dedicate a year of their lives to discovering other agricultural or productive realities and to carrying their experience and culture around the world. Instead of spending a year doing such activities as military service, the young of the food communities should be able to travel around the world to communities richer than their own, to poorer communities, to places where analogous forms of cultivation and production are practiced, and to the universities that teach agroecology.

The network of gastronomes could identify possible sources of finance for the journeys, and for their part, the communities, the chefs, and the universities could provide hospitality *free of charge* for a certain period to these young intellectuals of the earth. It will be necessary, of course, to draw up some rules, but the main principle is that of *giving freely*, of exchange without obligation, of being aware that these people are the conveyors of experiences that are *valuable* and that this value is the only price that is asked of them in exchange for their formative journeys.

Guaranteeing the *right to travel* (almost a duty for the young food producers and the gastronomes of the whole world) is another task for the network of gastronomes, weaving a system of values that will give to all the right of earthly citizenship, the right to be an active part of our "community of destiny."

4.2 The human values of the network: a new form of economy
The network of gastronomes will inevitably clash with individualism, the distances between cultures, and the distances
between economies. The principle of guaranteeing within it the
circulation of information, knowledge, products, and people is
one that *unites* people—in particular, those who can't even
dream of having these new experiences within the system of values that economic globalization is imposing. We must give economic value to other human values, in order to reconcile
individual advantage with that of the group.

The gift and *giving freely*: to rediscover the value of the gift
and of giving freely in a world like ours is to breathe life into the
system of new earthly citizenship that responsible gastronomes
desire. To make available one's own house, one's own food, one's
own culture is to open oneself to the world and to welcome it, in
the awareness that one *profits* by this. The profit is not merely
economic; it also consists of the certainty of increasing one's
knowledge, one's intellectual wealth, and one's potential for
development.

Free hospitality nourishes the system of unrestricted travel
and reintroduces an element of exchange that links together the
diversities in a creative force. The exchange does not claim to be
equal; the giving does not demand anything in return and does
not create any obligations, but is based on *confidence* in those
who share one's own community of destiny—on the confidence
that the destiny of a product or of economic resources has as
much *value* as what one gets back in *knowledge*, diversity or,
much more simply, in *friendship*.

What is the value of knowledge? It is incalculable, but its
worth becomes tangible in a network that is open to exchange,
that puts its resources into circulation. Knowledge is an inalien-
able right of all people, and it is nourished when this right is
shared among people. Knowledge is an opportunity that grows
and spreads in the complexity of the world. Everyone must be
able to participate; there must be no second-class or third-class
knowledge; every kind of knowledge has the same value, and can
become *currency*.

What is the value of saving, of sobriety? Wastage in the world has reached critical levels. It is unfair, and uneconomical—and not least because that which is wasted, if it were reused, would be an as yet unexploited resource. If consciences do not change in this regard, we will face increasing difficulties. We cannot ask everything of politics, we must begin to behave differently, starting with our own little everyday acts. What is *saved* must not become part of a logic of accumulation; what is saved can be *given*. Everyone must take on this responsibility, everyone can make their contribution. And in the vision of a network in which everyone is guaranteed the right to mobility and knowledge, the principle of *sobriety* becomes essential if resources are to be shared.

Gastronomy itself, before we forgot its more complex and important meanings, before it became a folkloristic exercise and was characterized by abundance and elitist wealth, endeavored to be an honest science practiced with moderation and sobriety. Still fundamental in this respect is the book by Bartolomeo Scappi, alias Il Platina, *De honesta voluptate* (On Honest Pleasure), where, alongside rules for eating well, there is an honest voluptuousness: this voluptuousness enhances pleasure, in responsible consumption, in the awareness that excess is always wrong, because it takes away richness and well-being from something or somebody, starting with ourselves. And excess is all the more wrong today, with the serious imbalances that weigh upon our staggering earth, imbalances which cause suffering to millions of farmers who work to produce food and to billions of people who are not able to eat as they could. Following a principle of *sobriety* is therefore the final (or principal) rule for the new gastronome, who joins a network for the common good: the gastronome who desires that his search for culinary pleasure, his atavistic need, should not deprive anyone else of the same pleasure—that of consuming a good, clean, and fair product, of which we may legitimately feel we are co-producers.

CONCLUSION

In conclusion, it is my hope that an ever-increasing number of people will choose to live seriously as new gastronomes—including representatives of the scientific world. Indeed, I would like to ask them to make a personal contribution: our aim is to make gastronomy a proper science, which will have to face the same difficulties of approach as, for example, the social sciences (the problem is epistemological), but which has all the prerequisites to become a subject of study at the university level and of research at even higher levels. Any discipline, if it does not remain closed within its own specialization, can lend some assistance to gastronomic science.

Besides, to say "gastronomic science" is rather like saying "the science of happiness." The chef Ferran Adrià, of all the people I asked for a definition of gastronomy, went to the heart of the matter. "Gastronomy is happiness!" he replied to me with a smile, his face tired and drawn after an evening's work in his phantasmagorical kitchen.

Happiness: so I would like to end by describing a scene I witnessed in Naples, at the San Carlo theater, in November 2003. The reader may try to visualize it.

It was during the award ceremony for the last Slow Food prize in defense of biodiversity (the event, of which this was the third occasion, was succeeded in 2004 by Terra Madre). The prize was a reward for all those people (about ten at each event) who had persuaded their communities to preserve a fragment of biodiversity. They were not great researchers, scientists, or figures of the institutional world; the prize was for farmers, fishermen, ordinary people, the "intellectuals of the earth." Each of them, in their various parts of the world, with their everyday work, made a small but significant contribution: they saved seeds, preserved and made profitable the production of threatened varieties or breeds, or strove to prevent the disappearance of something good, clean, and fair.

In Naples in 2003, the bestowing of the prize coincided with the world congress of Slow Food. We wanted the delegates from all over the world to be able to meet these heroes in person. For the award ceremony, which consecrated their status as champions of biodiversity, we chose a highly evocative place: the Teatro San Carlo.

Imagine the theater full of people from all over the world, wondrous to behold with its gilded stucco ornamentation, its red stalls, its walls which still echoed with all the music they had heard over the years, almost the entire history of Italian opera. One by one the prize-winners were called up onto the stage by Matthew Fort (a *Guardian* journalist) and the Italian actress Lella Costa. In each case, the reason for the award was read out in a language different from their own, and the microphone was available if they wanted to thank people, deliver a speech, or simply express their pride. It was a moving occasion, a truly unforgettable mixture of races, languages, and customs.

Eventually, it was the turn of Getulio Orlando Pinto Krahô, the chief of the Krahô community who began to grow the seeds of their native corn after recovering them from a germplasm bank in Brasilia.

So an Indian of the Brazilian *cerrado* was in Naples, thousands of kilometers away from his village; he had had the chance to familiarize himself with the city during the preceding days, wandering around with his serious, profound expression among the Slow Food delegates, on visits to the Campanian farmers, and at dinners in the local *osterie*. Although that year the late Neapolitan autumn had been mild, Getulio seemed not to be able to shake off the cold and was always wrapped up in a parka that someone had lent him. He seemed to examine everything and everyone, huddled up in that jacket which was several sizes too big. Everything was new to him, but he didn't seem in the least overawed; rather, he seemed slightly stiff, shy, aloof, transmitting a sense of dignity which fascinated everyone.

This vaguely humble attitude immediately disappeared when he was called up onto the stage of the San Carlo. After all, it was his moment, and it was to experience that precise instant that he had come all the way to Naples. He climbed the steps almost boldly, took the microphone with assurance and made a speech of thanks that left everyone open-mouthed.

This man, who together with his community had saved a seed and restored it to life, said: "I have no words to thank you; all this was unimaginable. I feel immensely happy, and when we Krahô are happy we express our feelings with a song. So please allow me to sing for you." And, taking the organizers of the pre-arranged ceremony completely by surprise, he sang a heart-rending tribal song for about three minutes, without any accompaniment. Few were unmoved; the silence in the hall was almost surreal. Those guttural sounds rang out thanks to the perfect acoustics of the theater, and the scene had something miraculous about it that sent a shiver down your spine.

On the same stage which had paid every honor to opera great Enrico Caruso, here was a Brazilian Indian singing simply because he was happy: he had been given a prize for saving a seed.

Those who witnessed that scene will never forget it, and in my opinion it was the greatest living expression of what gastronomic science—as a holistic vision of the world imbued with healthy human values—is and should be: a pure expression of happiness.

Perhaps it is here, in Getulio's voice at the San Carlo theater, in its simple but moving expression of joy, that we can find enough stimuli to make everyone, from the ordinary citizen to the distinguished scientist, accept the modest invitation that goes out from the pages of this book: to take part in creating a new gastronomy.

Finally, allow me to sign my name with pride in the following way:

I am a gastronome.

No, not a glutton with no sense of restraint whose enjoyment of food is greater the more plentiful and forbidden it is.

No, not a fool who is given to the pleasures of the table and indifferent to how the food got there.

I like to know the history of a food and of the place that it comes from; I like to imagine the hands of the people who grew it, transported it, processed it, and cooked it before it was served to me.

I do not want the food I consume to deprive others in the world of food.

I like traditional farmers, the relationship they have with the earth and the way they appreciate what is good.

The good belongs to everyone; pleasure belongs to everyone, for it is in human nature.

There is food for everyone on this planet, but not everyone eats. Those who do eat often do not enjoy it, but simply put gasoline into an engine. Those who do enjoy it often do not care about anything else: about the farmers and the earth, about nature and the good things it can offer us.

Few people know about the food they eat and derive enjoyment from that knowledge, a source of pleasure which unites all the people who share it.

I am a gastronome, and if that makes you smile, I assure you that it is not easy to be one. It is a complex matter, for gastronomy, though a Cinderella in the world of knowledge, is in fact a true science, which can open eyes.

And in this world of today it is very difficult to eat well, as gastronomy commands.

But there is a future even now, if the gastronome hungers for change.

APPENDIX

The complete text of the Manifesto on the Future of Food *can be viewed online at http://slowfood.com/about_us/eng/popup/ campaigns_future.lasso*

FROM THE MANIFESTO ON
THE FUTURE OF FOOD

Preamble: The failure of the industrialized agriculture model

The growing push toward industrialization and globalization of the world's agriculture and food supply imperils the future of humanity and the natural world. Successful forms of community-based local agriculture have fed much of the world for millennia, while conserving ecological integrity, and continue to do so in many parts of the planet. But they are being rapidly replaced by corporate-controlled, technology-based, monocultural, export-oriented systems. These systems of absentee ownership are negatively impacting public health, food quality and nourishment, traditional livelihoods (both agricultural and artisanal), and indigenous and local cultures, while accelerating indebtedness among millions of farmers and their separation from lands that have traditionally fed communities and families. This transition is increasing hunger, landlessness, homelessness, despair and suicides among farmers. Meanwhile, it is also degrading the planet's life-support systems, and increasing planet-wide alienation of peoples from nature and the historic, cultural, and natural connection of farmers and all other people to the sources of food and sustenance. Finally, it helps destroy the economic and cultural foundations of societies, undermines security and peace, and creates a context for social disintegration and violence.

Technological interventions sold by global corporations as panaceas for solving global problems of "inefficiency in small-scale production" and to supposedly solve world hunger have had exactly the opposite effect. From the Green Revolution, to the Biotech Revolution, to the current push for food irradiation, technological intrusions into the historic and natural means of local production have increased the vulnerability of ecosystems. They have brought pollution of air, water, and soil, and a new and spreading *genetic* pollution, from genetically modified organisms. These technology- and corporate-based monocultural systems seriously exacerbate the crisis of global warming by their heavy dependence upon fossil fuels and release of gases and other material. This latter fact alone—climate change—threatens to undermine the entire natural basis of ecologically benign agriculture and food preparation, bringing the likelihood of catastrophic outcomes in the near future. Moreover, industrial agriculture systems have certainly not brought increased efficiency in production, if one subtracts the ecological and social costs of this manner of production, and the immense public subsidies required. Nor do they reduce hunger; quite the opposite. They have, however, stimulated the growth and concentration of a small number of global agriculture giants who now control global production, to the detriment of local food growers, food supply and its quality, and the ability of communities and nations to achieve self-reliance in basic foods.

Already negative trends of the past half century have been accelerated by the recent rules of global trade and finance from global bureaucracies like the World Trade Organization (WTO), the World Bank, the International Monetary Fund, and the Codex Alimentarius, among others. These institutions have codified policies designed to serve the interests of global agribusiness above all others, while actively undermining the rights of farmers and consumers, as well as the ability of nations to regulate trade across their own borders or to apply standards appropriate to their communities. Rules contained in the Trade-Related Intellectual Property Rights Agreement (of the WTO), for example, have empowered global agricultural corporations to seize much of the world's seed supply, foods, and agricultural lands. The globalization of corporate-friendly patent regimes has also directly undermined indigenous and traditional *sui generis* rights of farmers, for example, to save seeds and protect indigenous varieties they have developed over millennia. Other WTO rules encourage export dumping of cheap subsidized agricultural products from industrial nations, thus adding to the immense difficulties of small farmers in poor countries to remain economically viable. And by invariably emphasizing export-oriented monocultural production, an explosion of long-distance trade in food products has had a direct correlation with increased use of fossil fuels for transport, thus further impacting climate, as well as the expansion of ecologically devastating infrastructure developments in indigenous and wilderness areas, with grave environmental consequences.

The entire conversion from local small-scale food production for local communities, to large-scale export-oriented monocultural production has also brought the melancholy decline of the traditions, cultures, and cooperative pleasures and convivialities associated for centuries with community-based production and markets, thereby diminishing the experience of direct food-growing, and the long celebrated joys of sharing food grown by local hands from local lands.

Despite all the above, there are many optimistic developments. Thousands of new and alternative initiatives are now flowering across the world to promote ecological agriculture, defense of the livelihoods of small farmers, production of healthy, safe, and culturally diverse foods, and localization of distribution, trade, and marketing. Another agriculture is not only possible; it is already happening.

For all these reasons and others, we declare our firm opposition to industrialized, globalized food production, and our support for this positive shift to sustainable, productive, locally adapted small-scale alternatives.

AFTERWORD

10 THINGS EVERY AMERICAN CAN DO TO STRENGTHEN OUR FOOD COMMUNITIES

- Join a local Slow Food convivium.

- Trace your food sources.

- Shop at a local farmers' market.

- Join a CSA (Community-Supported Agriculture).

- Invite a friend over to share a meal.

- Visit a farm in your area.

- Create a new food memory for a child! Let them plant seeds or harvest greens for a meal.

- Start a kitchen garden.

- Learn your local food history! Find a food that is celebrated as being originally from or best grown/produced in your part of the country.

For more information on Slow Food USA and to find your local chapter (convivium), visit www.slowfoodusa.org

BIBLIOGRAPHY

APOTEKER, ARNAUD. *L'invasione del pesce-fragola. Come viene manipo-lata la nostra alimentazione.* Rome: Editori Riuniti, 2000.

ARIÈS, PAUL. *Petit manuel anti-McDo à l'usage des petits et des grands.* Villeurbanne, France: Editions Golias, 1999.

————. *I figli di McDonald's. La globalizzazione dell'hamburger.* Bari: Dedalo, 2000.

ARTUSI, PELLEGRINO. *La scienza in cucina e l'arte di mangiar bene.* Torino: Einaudi, 1970.

BARBERIS, CORRADO. *Le campagne italiane dall'Ottocento a oggi.* Rome and Bari: Laterza, 1999.

BALL, A.S., TIM LANG, J.I.L. MORISON, and JULES PRETTY. "Farm Costs and Food Miles: An Assessment of the Full Cost," in *Food Policy*, v. 30, issue 1, September 2005, 1–19.

BEVILACQUA, PIERO. *La mucca è savia.* Rome: Donzelli, 2002.

BOLOGNA, GIANFRANCO, FRANCESCO GESUALDI, FAUSTO PIAZZA, and ANDREA SAROLDI. *Invito alla sobrietà felice.* Bologna: EMI, 2003.

BONAGLIA, FEDERICO and ANDREA GOLDSTEIN. *Globalizzazione e sviluppo.* Bologna: Il Mulino, 2003.

BOUDAN, CHRISTIAN. *Le cucine del mondo. Geopolitica dei gusti e delle grandi culture culinarie.* Rome: Donzelli, 2005.

BOURGUIGNON, CLAUDE and LYDIA BOURGUIGNON. *Il suolo, un patrimonio da salvare.* Bra, Italy: Slow Food Editore, 2004.

BOURRE, JEAN-MARIE. *La dietetica del cervello.* Milan: Sperling & Kupfer, 1992.

BOVÉ, JOSÉ and FRANÇOIS DUFOUR. *The World Is Not for Sale.* New York: Verso, 2002.

BRECHER, JEREMY and TIM COSTELLO. *Global Village or Global Pillage.* Cambridge, MA: South End Press, 1998.

BRILLAT-SAVARIN, JEAN-ANTHELME. *Physiologie du goût.* Paris: Flammarion, 1982.

CAPATTI, ALBERTO and MASSIMO MONTANARI. *La cucina italiana: Storia di una cultura.* Rome and Bari: Laterza, 1999.

CAPATTI, ALBERTO. *L'osteria nuova, una storia italiana del XX secolo.* Bra, Italy: Slow Food Editore, 2000.

CASSANO, FRANCO. *Modernizzare stanca.* Bologna: Il Mulino, 2001.

CENTRO NUOVO MODELLO DI SVILUPPO. *Guida al consumo critico.* Bologna: EMI, 2000.

CLOVER, CHARLES. *The End of the Line: How Over-fishing Is Changing the World and What We Eat.* New York: New Press, 2006.

CRANGA, FRANÇOISE and YVES CRANGA. *L'escargot.* Dijon: Les Editions du Bien Public, 1991.

DEB, DEBAL. *Industrial vs Ecological Agriculture.* New Delhi: Navdanya/Rfste, 2004.

Il dizionario di Slow Food. Bra, Italy: Slow Food Editore, 2002.

DOGANA, FERNANDO. *Psicopatologia dei consumi quotidiani.* Milan: Franco Angeli, 1993.

Encyclopédie des nuisances, I giocolieri del DNA nel pianeta dei creduloni.
    Turin: Bollati Boringhieri, 2000.
FISCHLER, CLAUDE. *L'onnivoro. Il piacere di mangiare nella storia e nella
    scienza*. Milan: Mondadori, 1990.
FLANDRIN, JEAN-LOUIS. *Il gusto e la necessità*. Milan: Il Saggiatore, 1994.
GESUALDI, FRANCESCO. *Manuale per un consumo responsabile*. Milan:
    Feltrinelli, 2002.
GIONO, JEAN. *Lettre aux paysans sur la pauverté et la paix*. Paris: Bernard
    Grasser, 1938.
GREW, RAYMOND. *Food in Global History*. Boulder, CO: Westview Press, 1999.
GRIMM, HANS-HULRICH. *L'imbroglio nella zuppa*. Bologna: Andromeda,
    1998.
HARDT, MICHAEL and ANTONIO NEGRI. *Empire*. Cambridge, MA:
    Harvard University Press, 2001.
HARRIS, MARVIN. *Good to Eat*. Long Grove, IL: Waveland, 1985.
HO, MAE-WAN. *Genetic Engineering Dream or Nightmare?*. New York:
    Continuum, 2000.
ILLICH, IVAN. *La convivialità*. Milan: Mondadori, 1974.
ISNENGHI, MARIO, ed. *I luoghi della memoria. Strutture ed eventi
    dell'Italia unita*. Rome and Bari: Laterza, 1997.
JAILLETTE, JEAN-CLAUDE. *Il cibo impazzito*. Milan: Feltrinelli, 2001.
JOLY, NICOLAS. *Le vin du ciel à la terre*. Paris: Editions Sang de la terre, 1997.
KIMBRELL, ANDREW, ed. *Fatal Harvest. The Tragedy of Industrial
    Agriculture*. Washington, D.C.: Island Press, 2002.
KLEIN, NAOMI. *No logo*. New York: Picador, 2002.
KUNDERA, MILAN. *Slowness*. New York: Harper, 1995.
LA CAMERA, FRANCESCO. *Sviluppo sostenibile. Origini, teoria e pratica*.
    Rome: Editori Riuniti, 2003.
LACROIX, MICHEL. *Le principe de Noé où l'Ethique de la sauvegarde*.
    Paris: Flammarion, 1997.
LACOUT, DOMINIQUE. *Le livre noir de la cuisine*. Paris: Jean-Paul Rocher
    Editeur, 2001.
LATOUCHE, SERGE. *Decolonizzare l'immaginario*. Bologna: EMI, 2004.
LAWRENCE, FELICITY. *Not on the Label*. New York: Penguin, 2004.
LEVI-STRAUSS, CLAUDE. *The Raw and the Cooked*. Chicago: University of
    Chicago Press, 1983.
LUTHER BLISSETT and CYRANO AUTOGESTITO DI ROVERETO.
    McNudo. Viterbo, Italy: Stampa Alternativa, 2001.
MANCE, EUCLIDES ANDRÉ. *La rivoluzione delle reti*. Bologna: EMI, 2003.
MERLO, VALERIO. *Contadini perfetti e cittadini agricoltori nel pensiero
    antico*. Milan: Jaca Book, 2003.
MONTANARI, MASSIMO. *Convivio Storia e cultura dei piaceri della tavola*.
    Rome and Bari: Laterza, 1991.
———. *Convivio Storia e cultura dei piaceri della tavola nell'età moderna*.
    Rome and Bari: Laterza, 1991.
———. *Convivio Storia e cultura dei piaceri della tavola nell'età contempo-
    ranea*. Rome and Bari: Laterza, 1992.
———, ed. *Il mondo in cucina. Storia, identità, scambi*. Rome and Bari:
    Laterza, 2002.
———. *Food Is Culture*. New York: Columbia University Press, 2006.

MORIN, EDGAR. *Introduzione a una politica dell'uomo*. Rome: Meltemi, 2000.
———. *Seven Complex Lessons in Education for the Future*. New York: UNESCO, 2001.
———. *Method*, vol. V. New York: Peter Lang, 1992.
NADOLNY, STEN. *The Discovery of Slowness*. Philadelphia: Paul Dry, 2005.
NANNI, ANTONIO. *Economia leggera. Guida ai nuovi comportamenti*. Bologna: EMI, 1997.
NISTRI, ROSSANO. *Dire, fare, gustare. Percorsi di educazione del gusto nella scuola*. Bra, Italy: Arcigola Slow Food, 1998.
ONFRAY, MICHEL. *La raison gourmande*. Paris: Grasset & Fasquelle, 1995.
ORTEGA CERDÁ, MIGUEL and DANIELA RUSSI. *Debito Ecologico*. Bologna: EMI, 2003.
PELT, JEAN-MARIE. *L'orto di Frankenstein*. Milan: Feltrinelli, 2000.
PERNA, TONINO. *Fair Trade*. Turin: Bollati Boringhieri, 1998.
PETRINI, CARLO. *Slow Food Revolution*. New York: Rizzoli International, 2006.
PONGE, FRANCIS. *Il partito preso delle cose*. Turin: Einaudi, 1979.
POULAIN, JEAN PIERRE. *Sociologies de l'alimentation*. Paris: PUF, 2002.
——— and EDMOND NEIRINCK. *Histoire de la cuisine et des cuisiniers*. Paris: Delgrave, 2004.
RIFKIN, JEREMY. *The Biotech Century*. New York: Tarcher, 1999.
RITZER, GEORGE. *The McDonaldization of Society*. Thousand Oaks, CA: Pine Forge Press, 2004.
———. *La religione dei consumi*. Bologna: Il Mulino, 2000.
SACHS, WOLFGANG, ed. *The Development Dictionary*. London: Zed Books, 1991.
SANSOT, PIERRE. *Du bon usage de la lenteur*. Paris: Manuels Payot, 1998.
SASSEN, SASKIA. *Globalizzati e scontenti. Il destino delle minoranze nel nuovo ordine mondiale*. Milan: Il Saggiatore, 2002.
SCHLOSSER, ERIC. *Fast Food Nation*. New York: Harper, 2001.
SEN, AMARTYA. *Development as Freedom*. New York: Anchor, 2000.
———. *La democrazia degli altri*. Milan: Arnoldo Mondadori, 2004.
SERVENTI, SILVANO and FRANÇOISE SABBAN. *La pasta, storia e cultura di un cibo universale*. Rome and Bari: Laterza, 2000.
SHIVA, VANDANA. *Monocultures of the Mind*. London: Zed Books, 1993.
———. *Stolen Harvest*. Cambridge, MA: South End Press, 2000.
———. *Vacche sacre e mucche pazze*. Rome: DeriveApprodi, 2001.
SMITH, JEFFREY M. *L'inganno a tavola*. Ozzano dell'Emilia, Italy: Nuovi Mondi Media, 2004.
SOROS, GEORGE. *The Crisis of Global Capitalism*. New York: PublicAffairs, 1998.
STIGLITZ, JOSEPH E. *Globalization and Its Discontents*. New York, London: W. W. Norton, 2002.
SÜSKIND, PATRICK. *Perfume*. New York: Vintage, 2001.
TAMINO, GIANNI and FABRIZIA PRATESI. *Ladri di geni*. Rome: Editori Riuniti, 2001.
Terra e Libertà / Critical Wine. Rome: DeriveApprodi, 2004.
TIGER, LIONEL. *The Pursuit of Pleasure*. Piscataway, NJ: Transaction, 2000.
VÉRON, JACQUES. *Popolazione e sviluppo*. Bologna: Il Mulino, 2001.
VERONELLI, LUIGI. *Breviario libertino*. Florence: Edizioni di Monte Vertine, 1984.

NOTES

1. See http://www.slowfoodfoundation.com/eng/premio/vincitori2003.lasso.
2. See the study by Carlo Bogliotti, on the site http://www.slowfoodfounda-tion.com/eng/premio/vincitori2002.lasso; or in the magazine *Slow Ark*, 35 (November 2002), p. 47.
3. Alessandro Monchiero, "Storie di ordinaria pazzia," *Slowine*, (June 2002).
4. Edgar Morin, *Method*, vol. V, (New York: Peter Lang, 1992), p. 227.
5. Jérôme Bindé, "Débattre des enjeux du futur," *Le Monde des Clubs Unesco*, VL (October 2000), quoted in Serge Latouche, *Decolonizzare l'immaginario* (Bologna: EMI, 2004), p. 38.
6. This is a concept from political economics: externalities of production occur when the production of an agent directly influences the production of another agent. There may be positive externalities and negative externalities—the former when there is a benefit due to the externality, the latter when there is a disadvantage. This kind of externality can create problems, because there are no markets for externalities (unless the government creates one), and therefore there are no prices for them.
7. Antonio Cianciullo, "Ambiente a rischio bancarotta," *La Repubblica*, 31 March 2005, p. 29.
8. Millennium Ecosystem Assessment, 2005, *Ecosystems and Human Well-being: Synthesis* (Island Press: Washington D.C., 2005), p. 1. See www.millenniumassessment.org.
9. Convention on Biological Diversity, Article 2, Use of Terms. See www.biodiv.org.
10. Millennium Ecosystem Assessment, *Synthesis*, p. 1.
11. Piero Bevilacqua, *La mucca è savia* (Rome: Donzelli, 2002), p. 22.
12. Debal Deb, *Industrial vs Ecological Agriculture* (New Delhi: Navdanya/Rfste, 2004), p. 4.
13. For more information on Portinari and Arcigola, see Carlo Petrini and Gigi Padovani, *Slow Food Revolution* (New York: Rizzoli International, 2006).
14. Massimo Montanari, *Food Is Culture* (New York: Columbia University Press, 2006), pp. 159–60.
15. Carlo Petrini, "Dialoghi sulla terra," *La Stampa*, 2 September 2004.
16. Jean-Anthelme Brillat-Savarin, *Physiologie du goût* (Paris: Flammarion, 1982).
17. Ibid.
18. Ibid., from the introduction by Jean-François Revel, p. 7.
19. Brillat-Savarin, *Physiologie du goût*, p. 57.
20. The following people participated in the first meeting of the Commission on the Future of Food: Debi Barker, co-director and chair of the Agricultural Committee of the International Forum on Globalization (IFG), USA; Marcello Buiatti, consultant on GMO issues to the Regional Council of Tuscany, director of the "Leo Pardi" Department of Animal and Genetic Biology, University of Florence, Italy; Arturo Compagnoni, World Board of the IFOAM, Italy; Christian Deverre, INRA (National Research

Institute on Agriculture), France; Peter Einarsson, European group of the IFOAM (International Federation of Biological Agriculture Movements), Swedish Ecological Farmers Association, Sweden; Elena Gagliasso, scientific coordinator for Lega Ambiente, lecturer in the Department of Philosophy and Epistemology of the University of Rome, Italy; Bernard Geier, represented by Louise Luttikholt, coordinator of IFOAM policies, Germany; Edward Goldsmith, author, founder and editor of *The Ecologist*, UK; Benny Haerlin, Foundation of Future Farming, former international coordinator of the anti-GMO campaign for Greenpeace, Germany; Colin Hines, also participating on behalf of Caroline Lucas, author of *Localisation: A Global Manifesto*, fellow, IFG, former head of the international economics unit of Greenpeace, UK; Vicky Hird, also participating on behalf of Tim Lang, policy director, Sustain: The Alliance for Better Food and Farming, UK; Frances Moore Lappe, author of *Diet for a Small Planet*, president of the Center for Living Democracy, USA; Jerry Mander, president of the board of the IFG, co-director of IFG, USA; Mark Ritchie, represented by Kristen Corselius, Institute for Agriculture & Trade Policy, USA; Peter Rosset, represented by Raj Patel, Food First, USA; Vandana Shiva, executive director of the Research Foundation for Science, Technology, and Ecology/Navdanya, India; Riccardo Simoncini, representing Yolanda Kakabadse, IUCN (The World Conservation Unit), scientific coordinator of the Aembach Project on Agriculture, Italy. The following did not participate in the Florence meeting but were included in all subsequent activities: Miguel Altieri, Gerald Assouline, Wendell Berry, Ronnie Cummins, Tewolde Egziabher, Bernward Geier, Zac Goldsmith, Andrew Kimbrell, Evelyn Fox Keller, Tim Lang, Caroline Lucas, Mark Ritchie, Anita Roddick, Peter Rosset, and Jan Douwe Van der Ploeg.

21. A complete digital copy can be viewed at www.pomonaitaliana.it.

22. Andrew Kimbrell, ed., *Fatal Harvest: The Tragedy of Industrial Agriculture* (Washington, D.C.: Island Press, 2002).

23. See Percy Schmeiser, *Davide vs.Golia*, in "Il cibo e l'impegno 2," *I quaderni di Micromega*, p. 123 (supplement to *Micromega*, no. 5, 2004).

24. Eric Schlosser, *Fast Food Nation* (New York: Harper, 2001), pp. 121–22.

25. Ibid., p. 127.

26. Wendell Berry, "The Pleasures of Eating," in *What Are People For?* (San Francisco: North Point Press, 1990).

27. From an interview with Miguel Altieri in Petrini, *Dialoghi sulla terra* (ibid., Note 15).

28. Marvin Harris, *Good to Eat* (Long Grove, IL: Waveland, 1985), p. 5.

29. Massimo Montanari, ed., *Il mondo in cucina: Storia, identità, scambi* (Rome and Bari: Laterza, 2002).

30. See Montanari, *Food Is Culture*.

31. See *Terra e Liberta'/ Critical Wine* (Rome: DeriveApprodi, 2004), p. 7.

32. Ibid., p. 9.

33. See Carlo Bogliotti at http://www.slowfoodfoundation.com/eng/premio/vincitori2003.lasso.

34. The founding of the medical school of Salerno probably dates back to the ninth century, but it was in the thirteenth century, under the influence of Frederick II's cultural program, that it rose to prominence, becoming the

principal center for the study and teaching of the medical sciences in the West, though in direct contact with, and strongly influenced by, the Arab tradition. The most well-known text produced by the Salerno school, the *Regimen sanitatis Salernitanum*, a popularizing medical manual in verse, was widely consulted for centuries.

35. Ugo Pollmer, "Voltar pagina," *Slow*, no. 34 (October 2002).
36. On the HACCP, see also Petrini and Padovani, *Slow Food Revolution*, p. 107.
37. Alberto Capatti and Massimo Montanari, *La cucina italiana: Storia di una cultura* (Rome and Bari: Laterza, 1999), p. 99.
38. Jean-Louis Flandrin, *Il gusto e la necessità* (Milan: Il Saggiatore, 1994).
39. Capatti and Montanari, *La cucina italiana*.
40. See Charles Clover, *The End of the Line: How Over-fishing Is Changing the World and What We Eat* (New York: New Press, 2006).
41. www.sciencedirect.com
42. Petrini, *Dialoghi sulla terra*. (ibid., Note 15).
43. Ibid.
44. Ibid.
45. Ibid.
46. Joseph E. Stiglitz, *Globalization and Its Discontents* (New York, London: W. W. Norton, 2002).
47. On these subjects, see for example Federico Rampini, *Il secolo cinese* (Milan: Mondadori, 2005).
48. Rossano Nistri, *Dire, fare, gustare. Percorsi di educazione del gusto nella scuola* (Bra, Italy: Arcigola Slow Food, 1998).
49. See www.unisg.it.
50. Alberto Capatti, personal communication.
51. Jean Giono, *Lettre aux paysans sur la pauvreté et la paix* (Paris: Bernard Grasset, 1938).
52. Agistment is an associative contract in the raising of livestock. There are three kinds of agistment: (1) simple, where one person, called the bailor, confers livestock on another person, the agistor, who takes upon himself the obligation to keep it, raise it, and process its products; (2) several, where the livestock is conferred by both people; (3) with conferment of pasture, where the livestock is conferred by the agistor and the bailor confers the land for pasture. In all three cases, it is always the agistor who is responsible for the keeping and raising of the livestock. The aim of this contract is to share the animals born during the contract, the increase in value of the livestock and the products. As far as the management of the business is concerned, that is the province of the bailor in the case of simple and several agistment, and of the agistor in the case of conferment of pasture.
53. Wendell Berry, personal communication.
54. Originally published by Oxford University Press, 1940, and reprinted by Rodale Press, 1979.
55. Nistri, *Dire, fare, gustare*, p. 21: "It was Galileo himself who took a negative view of the use of the senses in the application of the experimental method. He distinguished, as far as the quality of things is concerned, between those (imprecise and unreliable because unmeasurable) things which are linked with the sensations of the subject and those which are inherent in things themselves, because without them things would not even be conceivable.

Galileo called these latter qualities real accidents and held them to be the only ones that could lead to authentic knowledge, because they are expressible in mathematic terms, measurable in the true sense of the word."

56. From the Slow Food *Manifesto* (www.slowfood.it).
57. Ibid.
58. Franco Cassano, *Modernizzare stanca* (Bologna: Il Mulino, 2001), p. 154.
59. From an interview with Euzo Bianchi in Carlo Petrini, *Dialogo Sulla Terra* (ibid., Note 15).
60. Franco Cassano, *Modernizzare stanca* (Bologna: Il Mulino, 2001), p. 154.
61. In the speech that Lévi-Strauss gave at the awards ceremony of the Seventeenth International Catalunya Prizes in 2005; see *La Repubblica*, 15 June 2005.
62. Euclides André Mance, *La rivoluzione delle reti: L'economia solidale per un'altra globalizzazione* (Bologna: EMI, 2003), p. 25.
63. www.terramadre2004.org.
64. See *Terra Madre* (Bra, Italy: Slow Food, 2004).
65. Petrini, "Dialoghi sulla terra," no. 7, *La Stampa*, 2 August 2004.
66. Carlo Petrini (ed.), *Atlante delle grandi vigne di Langa* (Bra, Italy: Arcigola Slow Food, 1990), p. 230.